# "BLACK JACK" TO LOSE FAT

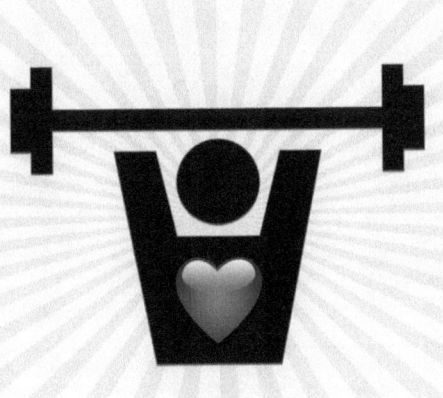

A guide to help
lower health risks
live a strong, active, and longer life!

**"CARPE DIEM"**
Seize the Day
Every Day!

## STACEY KARSERAS LPN

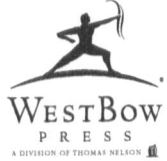

WestBow
PRESS
A DIVISION OF THOMAS NELSON

WestBow Press books may be ordered through booksellers or by contacting:

WestBow Press
A Division of Thomas Nelson
1663 Liberty Drive
Bloomington, IN 47403
www.westbowpress.com
1-(866) 928-1240

Because of the dynamic nature of the Internet, any web addresses or links contained in this book may have changed since publication and may no longer be valid. The views expressed in this work are solely those of the author and do not necessarily reflect the views of the publisher, and the publisher hereby disclaims any responsibility for them.

Any people depicted in stock imagery provided by Thinkstock are models, and such images are being used for illustrative purposes only.

Certain stock imagery © Thinkstock.

ISBN: 978-1-4497-1512-0 (sc)
ISBN: 978-1-4497-1507-6 (e)

Library of Congress Control Number: 2011926195

Printed in the United States of America

WestBow Press rev. date: 4/1/2011

# Credits

Concorde Career Institute CNA

The School of Fitness and Nutrition

Erwin Technical Center School of Nursing LPN

WestBow Press, a division of Thomas Nelson Publishing

Images from Thinkstock®

# Dedications

I dedicate this book to:

My father, who suffered with heart disease and other health problems due to an intake of unhealthy nourishment choices and lack of consistent physical fitness. The heart attack, quadruple coronary bypass surgery, sleep apnea, cardiac arrhythmia, and chronic pain weren't enough to convince him that he needed to change his lifestyle if he wanted to survive. My father tried several diets; at times, he leisurely played golf. Unfortunately, diets and lack of physical fitness place the body at risk for health problems, and the body requires physical resistance to thrive. We miss him dearly.

Next is a coworker that had an unsuccessful gastric bypass surgery and passed away within twenty-four hours of the surgery due to a blood clot that dislodged from the wall of an artery and traveled to one of her lungs.

All of my patients who I thought were in denial or naive, but I found out that they were just uneducated about their own health.

My family, especially my mother Sandy, who is my main support system I thank and love all of you.

# Contents

# Introduction:
# Over fat = Unhealthy

The saying "You are what you eat" is true, and Richard Simmons really does have that much energy. So can you! When each of us makes unhealthy nourishment choices and does not incorporate consistent physical resistance training in our lives, then we do not produce an adequate amount of oxygenated blood that the heart, brain, and body need, thus increasing the risks for health problems.

Even if we are not lazy, we appear to be lazy. Too much fat places stress on the organs, muscles, joints, and bones. The lack of activity also creates health problems, especially as we grow older, retire, and are usually more sedentary. Lack of mobility equals lack of motility, and even a simple bowel obstruction could have the potential to result in death.

An active or physically fit lifestyle is easier to achieve if the changes are gradual but consistent. Choose healthy nourishment choices to increase the metabolism and decrease hunger, cravings, bingeing, anxiety, depression, and other health problems.

# Be a Winner with "Black Jack"

Have you ever started a diet, purchased all the proper foods and beverages, and by day two you are ready to throw in the towel and eat a gallon of ice cream? Well, those days are over! It is time to eat to live and not live to eat. I love to cook and I love to eat, but I also would rather live longer and be free of pain and illness. With moderation as the key, enter the world of "Black Jack"—a combination of healthy nourishment choices and consistent resistance training to lose fat, become strong, feel great, and maybe even look younger! Everyone deserves to feel good and be able to move about gracefully, not waddle. Stop stepping up to the table just to fold! Flip the cards and win with "Black Jack" and "Carpe Diem" (seize the day)! Allow yourself one day a week, for example, game day or family day, that you can relax, eat in moderation, and enjoy your favorite foods and beverages without feeling guilty. There will not be any guilt with this new way of life because you are your own personal trainer. Use this book as a guide to getting your body and groove back!

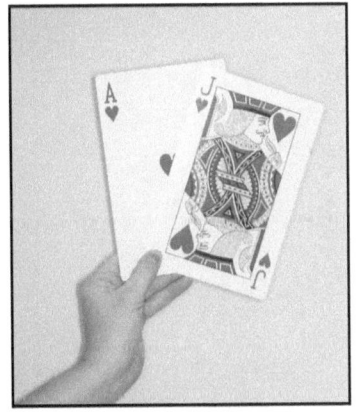

Don't be fooled anymore by infomercials that use people who train for hours with heavy resistance before advertising their product. In order to achieve the physique that they have, you have to resistance train, and that is exactly what they do. I do not know many people who can shake a weight for one minute, not to mention six minutes! Many personal trainers have been overweight and over fat at one time in their life, and they have conquered the fat demon. You can too! So, again, "Carpe Diem"—seize the day! It is *your* turn to *win* with "Black Jack" 21!

One week = 168 hours

Three "Black Jack" sessions = two hours

Leaving 166 hours and plenty of time for the rest of your life so stop finding time to be lazy; use that time to become active and alive.

Use "Black Jack" 21 three times a week for the rest of your life. If time doesn't allow the whole session, then perform ten minutes. Any length of time is better than none!

# Definitions

In this chapter I define all of the terms that are mentioned in the book.

<u>ADLs</u>:  Activities of daily living

<u>Advance directive</u>: includes many types of legal documentation that is enforced by an individual regarding health and financial matters

> Living will is a legal document that is enforced if an individual is unable to make medical decisions

> Health care surrogate (HCS) is a legal document that appoints another individual to make healthcare decisions on someone else's behalf

> Power of attorney (POA) is a legal document that appoints an individual to make financial decisions on someone else's behalf

> Do not resuscitate (DNR) is a legal document that states an individuals wishes in case of an emergency regarding life saving measures

<u>Aerobic</u>: A type of exercise that uses oxygen and usually burns calories. Examples: swimming, walking, dancing/aerobics, bicycling

<u>Anaerobic</u>: A type of exercise that does not use oxygen. Example: resistance training

<u>Anticoagulants</u>: Products that thin the blood and may increase the risk for bleeding

<u>Antihypertensive medications or supplements</u>: Products that lower the pressure in the blood

<u>Artery</u>: A tube that carries blood at a high pressure from the heart to the body

<u>Atrophy</u>: Stiffness or immobility of extremities and organs

<u>Blood clots</u>: Particles from tissue, cholesterol, infected material; tumors, fat cells, bone marrow, air, and nitrogen that break off of the artery wall and can become dislodged, increasing the potential to travel to the heart, lungs, or brain

<u>Blood sugar</u>: The amount of sugar in the blood

<u>Bone</u>: The skeletal structure of the body, where calcium is produced. Bones can have small, medium, or large structure.

<u>Capillary</u>: The webbed network between the arteries and veins where the interchange of oxygen, carbon dioxide, and nutrients takes place

<u>Carbohydrate</u>: Energy compounds that we gain from nourishment

<u>Cardiologist</u>: A physician who specializes in cardiovascular conditions

<u>Casein</u>: A nutrient in milk and cheese that helps build muscle because it prepares the body to use more calcium

<u>Contraindications</u>: Risks that may occur if more than one medication or supplement is taken at one time

<u>Diet</u>: The choices that a person makes to nourish the body

<u>Endorphins</u>: Neurotransmitters that aid in regulating the heart, hormone function, perception of pain, emotions, and motivation

<u>Gait</u>: How steady a person is on his/her own feet. An unsteady gait may require a cane, walker, crutches, wheelchair, etc.

<u>Glycemic index value</u>: The value that a food is given depending on how much sugar it contains. Levels range from low ($\leq$55) to medium (56–69) to high ($\geq$70).

<u>Hypervitaminosis</u>: High levels of vitamins in the blood

<u>IBS</u>: Irritable bowel syndrome; bouts of constipation and diarrhea

<u>Immunocompromised</u>: A decreased ability to fight viral or bacterial infections or cancers

<u>Inflammation</u>: Swelling

Injury: A semi permanent or permanent dysfunction that prevents full range of motion in a particular area of the body

Insulin: Regulates carbohydrates, fats, proteins, and metabolism and is produced by the pancreas

Lipid lowering agents: Products that lower cholesterol like triglycerides

Melatonin: A hormone that assists with sleep

Metabolism: The energy produced by the body from our nourishment choices and level of daily activity

Mobility: The ability to move

Motility: Spontaneous movement. The bowels need motility to occur properly, and this is called peristalsis.

Muscle: A tissue that has the capabilities of lengthening and thickening; it attaches to the bone.

Muscle protein synthesis: The ability of amino acids to repair and reinforce muscle fibers while boosting the strength in the bones and muscles, thus increasing flexibility, HGH (human growth hormone, i.e., the fat-burning hormone), and the metabolism

NSAIDS: Nonsteroidal anti-inflammatory drug products that thin the blood and may increase the risk for bleeding

Obesity: The state of being over fat, placing stress on the bones, muscles, joints, and organs of the body

Oral diabetic medications or supplements: Products that lower the blood sugar levels in the blood

Osteopenia: The beginning of osteoporosis (decreased bone density). Osteoporosis can cause curvature of the spine; weak bones increase the risk of bone fractures

Pain: An unpleasant sensation caused by an injury, inflammation, or a physical or psychological situation

PCP: Primary care physician

<u>Plaque</u>: An accumulation of plaque that appears in the artery wall due to high cholesterol and triglyceride levels in the blood, high blood pressure, stress, and/or smoking

<u>Satiety</u>: The state of feeling satisfied after eating

<u>Scale</u>: A device that can measure a person's body weight

<u>Side effects</u>: Reactions that may occur after taking a product

<u>Skin</u>: The major organ of the body. It is lubricating, self-regenerating, and repairing itself all the time. New cells and tissue growth are induced by vitamin D (i.e., the sunshine vitamin).

<u>Stomach</u>: The pouch that holds nourishment. It holds approximately 1.75L (liters).

<u>Stretch marks</u>: Striated marks that appear on the skin when the skin is stretched

<u>Tonicity</u>: How toned a muscle appears

<u>Triglyceride</u>: A component of cholesterol; high levels cause health risks, such as metabolic syndrome, obesity, diabetes, thyroid diseases, kidney problems, heart disease, and arteriosclerosis. Some medications, foods with high GI levels, and alcoholic beverages can also raise these levels.

<u>Vein</u>: A vessel that carries blood from the capillaries toward the heart

# Health Problems

In this chapter I include the health problems that are described in the book and several options that may decrease the risks.

Acid reflux: Irritants that may include medication, foods, and beverages; may cause indigestion

Allergies: Hypersensitivity to certain allergens, medications, or seasonal, environmental, or chemical irritants

Anemia: Low levels of iron in the blood

Anxiety: A response to a threat or danger, causing a fight or flight response

Arthritis: Inflammation of a joint due to the natural aging processes, repetitive movements, and/or too much weight bearing on a joint

CABG: Coronary artery bypass graft, wherein a coronary artery is bypassed and grafted onto another artery

Cancer: An internal or external malignant growth that can invade the body in various forms

Cardiovascular and respiratory disease: Disease of the heart and lungs

Carotid artery disease: Disease of the carotid arteries on each side of the neck that supply oxygenated blood to the brain

Celiac disease: Intolerance to products that contain gluten

Depression: The state of feeling sad, unworthy, anxious, and tired, lacking the ability to concentrate

Headache: Pain in the head, face, sinus, or neck

<u>Hyperglycemia</u>: High blood sugar levels, which increase the risk for type 2 diabetes

<u>Hypertension</u>: High blood pressure. This is a heart problem and increases the risk for a heart attack. Common culprits are sodium (from high-sodium diets) and lack of physical fitness.

<u>Hyperthyroid</u>: An overactive hormone production of iodine, which may present itself in goiters and nodules (growths)

<u>Hypoglycemia</u>: Low blood sugar levels, which increase the risk for type 1 diabetes

<u>Hypotension</u>: Low blood pressure, which increases the risk for a stroke

<u>Hypothyroid</u>: An underactive hormone production in the thyroid

<u>Sleep apnea</u>: An obstruction of the airway that usually occurs while sleeping, which includes periods without breathing; may cause tiredness during waking hours

<u>Stress</u>: Physical, psychological, and social situations that threaten a person's well-being or safety, resulting in a fight or flight response

<u>Stroke</u>: The event that occurs if oxygenated blood does not reach the brain

<u>Type 1 diabetes</u>: The inability of the pancreas to produce and secrete insulin, increasing the risk of insulin dependence (IDDM or insulin dependent diabetes mellitus)

<u>Type 2 diabetes</u>: Too much sugar in the blood. A person may need something to lower the blood sugar levels, making a person oral dependent or non insulin dependent (NDDM or non insulin dependent diabetes mellitus) In time, a person who is a type 2 diabetic due to the inability of the pancreas to produce insulin may become a type 1 diabetic. Type 2 diabetes is usually acquired from too much sugar in the diet, and sugar is usually the cause of obesity.

# My Experiences Working in Health Care

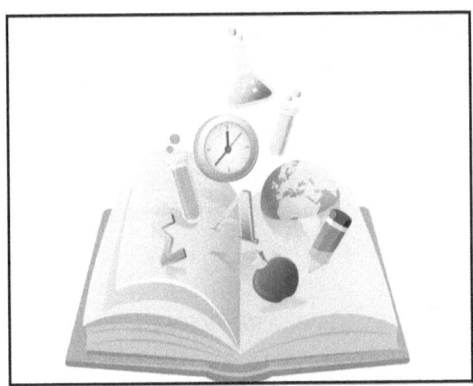

During the last twenty-five years, I have worked in health care, and I have carried too much fat on my body, just like most of my co-workers. I finally came to the conclusion that we are not very good role models for our patients, and if we are not careful, we will become the patient. The shifts are sometimes brutal. A meal includes grabbing something fast and eating it fast. By the time our shift is over, we are usually hungry again, and the last thing we want to do is exercise.

I took care of many patients, some of whom had their sternum sawed in half to have heart surgery, just like my father; and many patients who had successful and unsuccessful surgeries, including cosmetic surgery and many others. I observed many of them, and I concluded that there isn't a magic pill, magic diet, or magic surgery that will get us into shape or improve our health. In addition, the best chance that we have at achieving this is with healthy nourishment choices and a regular resistance training exercise program.

The body is composed of three things:
1. Bones or the skeleton, which supports and frames the body
2. Muscles, which give us strength
3. Fat, which is necessary for insulating, cushioning, and protecting the organs of the body from trauma

The state of being too fat or obese places stress on the bones, joints, muscles, and organs of the body, and causes the heart to pump harder and faster. It makes the capillaries less efficient, which increases the risk for high blood pressure, other health problems, medications, and surgeries. You are your own personal trainer. Three approaches that increase the chance for long-term success and fat loss are: 1) throw away the scale, because we are not focusing on weight, 2) learn the definition of the word "diet," and 3) decrease the capacity of your stomach the natural way.

The stomach holds approximately 1.75 liters, and each time that we overeat or stuff ourselves, the stomach stretches and expands to allow us to eat more the next time. Many patients who are survivors of a gastric augmentation have been able to stretch their stomach again and now live with eating and vomiting many times every day. In addition, this places them at a higher the risk for more gastrointestinal as well as other health problems and additional surgeries.

Over time, I realized that many patients are not in denial or naïve; they are just uneducated about their own health. Like my father, who didn't understand that an all-protein diet was supposed to be lean protein and not protein full of fat like a half pound of bacon! It is important that we all learn about our health and the risks that may occur if we live an unhealthy, sedentary lifestyle. We must teach our younger generation about health and be good role models; I see too many pediatric patients suffering from cardiovascular disease, and it is disheartening.

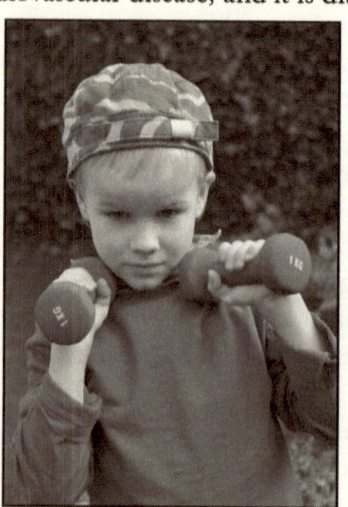 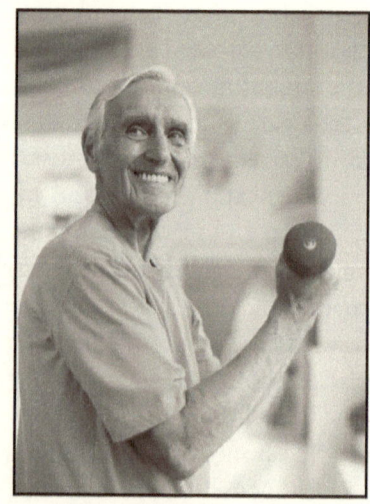

Become active as a family! Anyone over the age of four can train with resistance, and everyone will reap the benefits that being active can provide. "Black Jack" 21 includes a five-minute warm-up to increase the heart rate and oxygen level, a thirty-minute, twenty-one resistance training exercise circuit, and a five-minute cool down to allow the blood to circulate back into the body.

This workout program will require effort, but the effort becomes easier with each session. Each session will increase your strength, endorphins, and level of energy. You will also stabilize your blood sugar and mood levels, decreasing aches and pains.

The key is to start gradually and incorporate healthy nourishment choices daily that will fuel the body. Slowly add regular exercise, such as marching in place for a few minutes and moving the arms up and down to increase the heart rate and oxygen level. By making gradual changes, you increase your chance for long-term success.

# What Is Fat?

Fat is adipose tissue, which is the accumulation or expansion of fat cells. The main purpose of fat is to cushion and protect the major organs of the body. Too much fat will compromise our organs, causing crowding as the fat and organs compete for room inside the body, increasing the risk for health problems. Fat cells also contain a protein that has the potential to cause inflammation and chronic pain. Some people have more fat cells than others, and once you become fat it, is harder to lose fat. You did not become fat overnight, and over time, fat loss can be achieved gradually. The order that fat is added to the body will be the order in which it is removed from the body, you cannot spot train a specific area, but you can increase lean muscle mass all over the body for maximum fat-burning results in all areas of the body that have extra fat! By this method, you can achieve or maintain the fat-free body you have always desired!

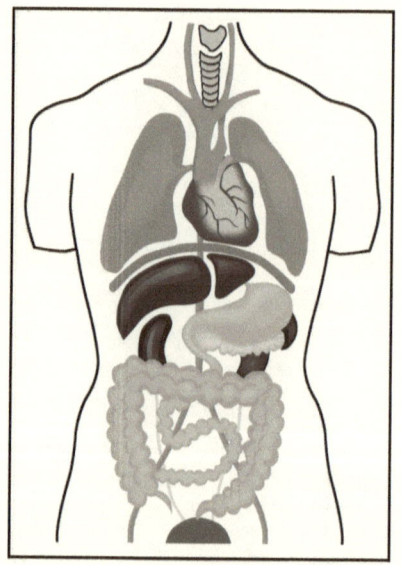

Have reasonable expectations and take one day at a time—or better yet, take one meal/snack at a time for long-term success. Stop allowing fat to hold you back.

# How to Burn Fat

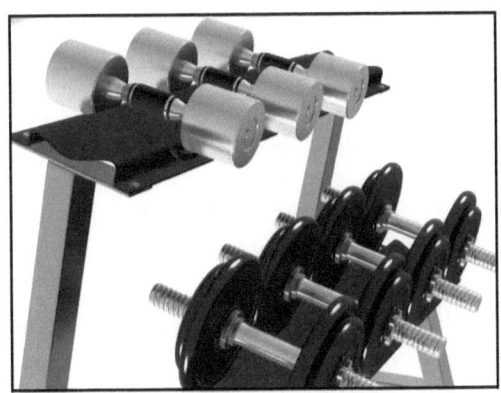

The only way to burn fat is to increase lean muscle mass and increase the heart rate. The best way to increase lean muscle mass is with resistance training, and this can include several types of resistance. These types include the body's resistance, bands, cables, pulleys, nautilus machines, free weights, and dumbbells. Dumbbells are versatile, portable, and the least expensive type of resistance to provide maximum results.

The amount of resistance used is determined by how many repetitions are performed. When a muscle is slightly stressed toward the last exercise or repetition of a set, but the correct range of motion is achieved at all times.

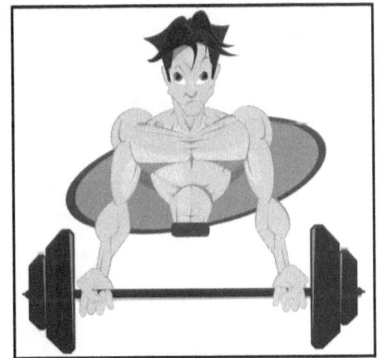

The old motto "No pain, no gain" no longer applies. Three important things to avoid while resistance training includes:

1. Injury
2. Exhaustion
3. Unnecessary muscle soreness

Do not compromise the proper form of an exercise in order to lift the weight through the full range of the muscle or joint called range of motion.

If the resistance is too heavy, don't lift it. The recovery time between resistance training sessions should be thirty-six to forty-eight hours. If your muscles are sore twenty-four hours after resistance training, then the resistance is too heavy. Feel free to perform cardiovascular or aerobic exercises or recreational activities after resistance training or on the alternate days for added benefits.

When the body becomes strong and free of fat, it is easier to perform recreational or leisure activities. Such a state of fitness decreases the risk for pulled muscles, bone fractures, and disabilities due to unnecessary injuries.

Bone density decreases as we age. Resistance training strengthens the muscles, increases calcium production, and strengthens the bones, thus increasing bone density.

Fad diets and weight loss gimmicks that promote fast weight loss place the body at risk for losing lean muscle mass, bone density, water weight, and tonicity.

Weight loss is different than fat loss. Weight loss from muscle, bone, or water increases health problems. But fat loss by increasing lean muscle mass and bone density increases health benefits.

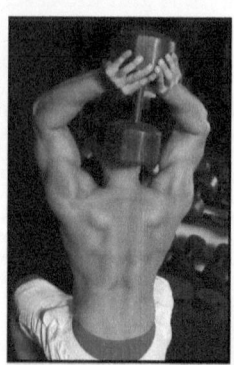 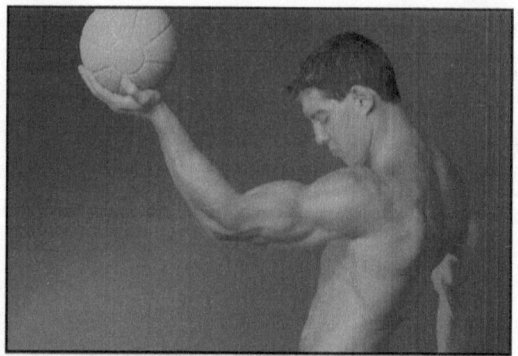

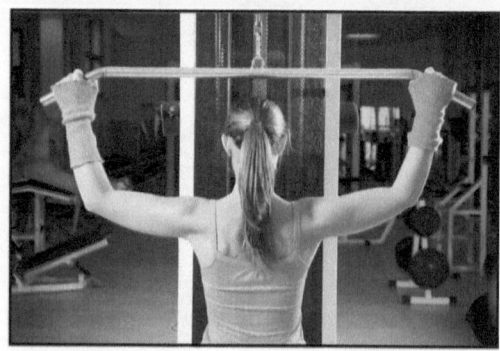

# Why Do We Get Hungry?

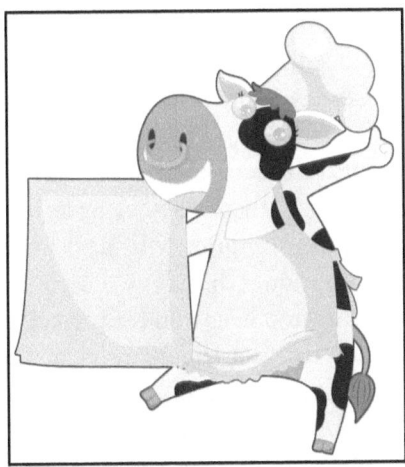

Hunger is controlled by blood sugar levels. Blood glucose is the amount of sugar in the blood. Carbohydrates that contain sugar will have a higher glycemic index value. If we eat too many carbohydrates and our energy storage is full, then the additional carbohydrates that are eaten will be stored in fat cells. Too much sugar in the blood may predispose a person for obesity and type 2 diabetes. Foods with high glycemic index values that are eaten every day in combination with a nonphysical lifestyle predispose a person to so many health problems.

Foods that seem healthy may actually sabotage fat loss. Sugar is hidden in many types of products, such as beverages, sauces, gravies, condiments, dressings, ice cream, frozen yogurt, bread, and yes, vegetables, especially potatoes, corn, carrots, and peas.

Our blood sugar reacts to the amount of starch that a product contains. Usually the more starch in a food, the more sugar an item will contain and the higher the glycemic index value will be. Blood sugar levels fall or drop every four hours or so depending on an individual's health. It is important to fuel the body like a car, always providing fuel to spark it up and keep it moving. We must feed the body frequently during waking hours to prevent hunger and low blood sugar levels or crashes. Proper feeding will decrease the risks for lethargy, headaches, irritability, shaking, and low productivity. This is the reason that it is important to eat after you awaken from a long sleep: to kick the metabolism into gear like a spark plug on a car. The car will not start if it doesn't have a spark.

Fueling the body frequently with healthy choices will stabilize blood sugar levels and minimize cravings and binges. Bingeing causes a fast spike in the blood sugar, triggering the pancreas to secrete insulin, which lowers the blood sugar back to normal over time. This can lead to the inability of the pancreas to produce insulin effectively when needed. This type of instability is what causes a person to crave sugar and starch, leading to another binge.

To lose fat or prevent fat, reduce enriched bread, sugar, pasta, potatoes, rice, corn, carrots, and peas. These choices have higher glycemic index values, so reducing their consumption will help to stabilize blood sugar and lower caloric consumption. Choices that have lower glycemic index values provide more energy and keep you feeling full or satisfied longer in between meals or snacks. It is not the quantity of the carbohydrate, but the quality that is important. The secret is to eat before you are hungry, to prevent cravings and decrease the chance of bingeing.

Incorporate healthy nourishment choices daily and do not avoid everything at one time. Remember, everything in moderation, so be mindful of portions and serving sizes.

# What Should We Eat?

There are many forms of sugar: glucose, sucrose, and fructose. Glucose is sugar and our main source of energy; it is the type of carbohydrate that raises blood sugar, and too much sugar is usually the reason for being fat.

Simple carbohydrates include fruits that contain natural sugar but have a lower GI value and high fiber contents and will keep you feeling full longer. Complex carbohydrates higher in starch that have higher glycemic index values include rice, legumes, and root vegetables, like potatoes and are the items that you want to keep to a minimum. Since these types of foods break down easily, you are left with pure glucose, which raises the blood sugar levels quickly if eaten with fat. You will be hungry again soon after eating such foods.

Hidden sugars are found in fibrous, non-digestible carbohydrates, such as fruits, grains, and leaves of vegetables. Two other forms of sugar are sucrose and fructose. Sucrose is table sugar and is also used as a preservative. It is found in baked goods and most junk food, spiking blood sugar levels and then resulting in a crash due to unstable blood sugars. Fructose doesn't spike blood sugar levels, but after traveling through the intestines and liver, the fructose is converted to glucose and stored as energy or fat. Fiber is composed of bundles of sugar molecules but has no effect on blood sugar. Fiber slows down the absorption of starch into your bloodstream and keeps you satisfied longer. Good examples of these food choices with lower glycemic index values are avocados, citrus fruits (tangerines and oranges are great choices) apples, and prunes.

Try to incorporate high-quality protein with every meal, such as eggs, cheese, plain or vanilla Greek yogurt, natural peanut butter/old fashioned peanut butter, nuts, fish, shellfish, and lean pork, beef, or poultry. Eat lean protein one hour before a resistance training session or within thirty minutes afterward for optimum muscle-building and repairing benefits.

Eat healthy fats in moderation. Examples include extra virgin olive oil, butter, natural nuts, seeds, olives, full fat sour cream, regular salad dressings, coconut, and avocados. Eat low-starch or low GI valued vegetables, such as asparagus, artichokes, brussel sprouts, broccoli, cucumbers, mushrooms, onions, peppers, spinach, tomatoes, turnips, and zucchini. Limit bread, especially if the first ingredient includes the word "enriched." Drink as much water as possible, making this your primary means of hydration. Drink coffee and tea in moderation. Be mindful about the sweeteners used. Artificial sweeteners have health risks, increase hunger, and may be precursors for type 2 diabetes. The lower the fat content that a product has, the higher its sugar content will be. For example, skim milk and 1 percent milk have more sugar than 2 percent or whole milk.

Try to eat food that is as close to its natural state as possible. For example, unsalted nuts are better for you than processed nuts, and you can make your own homemade nuts (see nut recipe in a later chapter).

The daily recommended amount of sugar is forty grams. Each sugar cube, sugar packet, or teaspoon of sugar contains sixteen calories and four grams of sugar.

The recommended daily allowance of sodium/salt is 2,300 mg.

## Glycemic Index/GI

This chart will show the amount of sugar or starch that a product has by the Glycemic Index Value it contains. The higher the number the faster the blood sugar levels will be increased.

### *Low GI (55 or less)*

fructose and products low in carbohydrates, most fruits especially avocados and vegetables, whole grains, legumes, milk, eggs, nuts, meat

### *Medium GI (56–69)*

sucrose, table sugar, sweet potato, basmati rice, whole wheat products, products with preservatives, baked goods, junk foods

### *High GI (70 or above)*

glucose, white bread, most white rices, cornflakes, most breakfast cereals with sugar added, baked potatoes and potato products, e.g., french fries, watermelon

# When Should We Eat?

The best time to eat is before you become hungry. Since your blood sugar falls every three to four hours, the body should be fueled accordingly to prevent spikes, crashes, hunger, headaches, cravings and low metabolism. Eat soon after awakening and frequently during waking hours to stabilize blood sugar. Resistance training will burn fat for a full twenty-four hours after a session, so as long as you are increasing lean muscle mass, you can eat anytime. It wouldn't make sense to suggest to a person that works the night shift to stop eating after 9:00 p.m. because this is probably the time this person is ready for a snack or a meal. The body is made up of 60 percent water, and this amount increases with the nourishment choices we make, especially if the choices contain sodium/salt or preservatives. Drink plenty of water before a meal or snack because hunger is sometimes mistaken for dehydration. Eat protein one hour before a workout and within thirty minutes afterward for maximum muscle-building and repairing benefits.

# How to Treat Your Body with Respect

Incorporate resistance training and healthy nourishment choices every day for long-term fat loss. The body thrives on the right kind of resistance, and it doesn't take long to feel and notice the benefits. The body produces hormones and neurotransmitters, and the amounts or effects increase with physical activity, stabilizing mood levels and decreasing pain. When the body is stable, strong, and free from pain, we breathe and sleep better, we become more productive, and we feel and look ten years younger.

Before you take vitamins, minerals, or any other supplements, have your blood levels checked because too much of any of these products can do more harm than good. Refer to hypervitaminosis in the chapter on definitions.

Gradual changes will lead to long-term success, so throw away the scale and be more concerned with how you feel and look. Healthy people usually look healthy and are happy because they feel good. Stop placing yourself at risk for being the next guinea pig for the next fad diet or miracle cure.

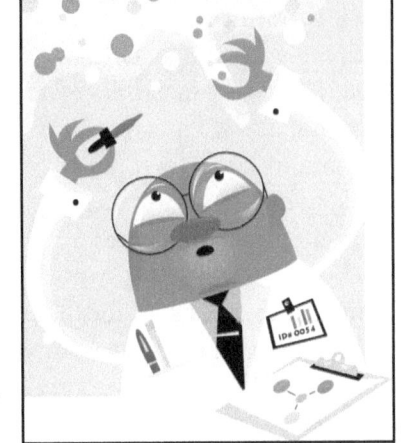

The reason people increase their risks of death revolves around mobility. Lack of mobility equals lack of motility, thereby causing problems in the muscles, joints, bones, organs, and bodily functions. A simple bowel obstruction has the potential to cause death for many people, especially the elderly.

I always wondered why the word diet sounds and looks like the word "die." That is why it is important to always remain active and agile.

# Finding Time to Exercise

The more you enjoy your workout session, the better the chance that you will do it again and again and again! After a long day at work, the last thing someone wants to do is work out. But if you were able to work out to your own music, music video, favorite show, or movie, the chances would be greater that you would want to work out!

I have created a resistance training program that will fit into anyone's schedule. It is one the whole family over the age of four can perform together. "Black Jack" 21 is a resistance training program taking twenty-one resistance training exercises and incorporating two sets of fifteen repetitions each, performed in a circuit without a rest in between exercises or sets. I incorporate a five-minute warm-up and a five-minute cool down. This workout takes approximately forty minutes three times a week and equals about two

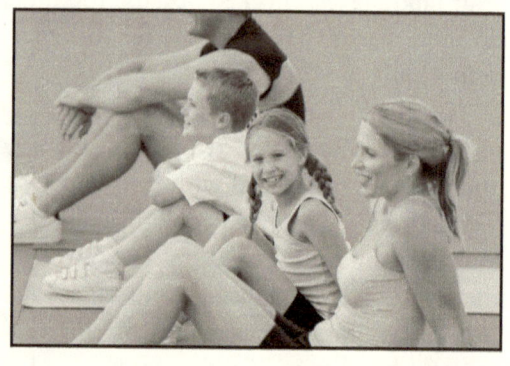

hours. Each week has 168 hours, so 168 hours − 2 hours = 166 hours. Each session takes the same amount of time that it takes to order a pizza or buy fast food. This workout is quick, and in no time, the two sets of the twenty-one "Black Jack" exercises are completed at your own pace and time. Drink plenty of water before, during, and after each session to prevent dehydration. Stop if a rest is required and wipe the sweat from your brow when necessary.

Since this workout program is easy and fast, it doesn't take long to feel and see results. I spent hours on my treadmill power walking for almost two years before I realized that the fat was not going to disappear until I increased lean muscle mass all over the body. Once I did that, then it literally melted away. I feel energized afterward and not tired or exhausted as I felt after power walking ten miles a week. The benefits from resistance training will change your life, increasing the oxygen in the blood and improving the heart, lungs, brain, and bodily functions.

I recommend a dumbbell because it is versatile, portable, and inexpensive. It also takes up the least amount of room. I work out in a room with a TV and radio because I enjoy my sessions more if I have something that will slightly distract me while I perform "Black Jack" 21. Like many of you, I tried many fad diets and diet pills. I even thought about weight loss augmentation surgeries, but I have a very low pain tolerance. I wanted to decrease my pain, not increase it, so I decided to get moving, start living, and get off my rear end. I look forward to resistance training three days a week, and I no longer make excuses for being tired or feeling bad.

# The Best Time to Exercise

Always seek the advice of a physician before beginning any program that alters nourishment and includes exercise. Then the best time to exercise is approximately four hours after eating because the blood sugar levels are low at that time and this will promote optimum fat-burning results. Also at that time, the carbohydrate stores are low, and HGH (human growth hormone) is at its highest potential.

Do not work out until at least one hour after awakening because it usually takes this long for the spinal fluid to lubricate the spinal cord to prevent spinal injuries. Aerobic activity is more beneficial if performed after resistance training or on alternate days between "Black Jack" 21sessions.

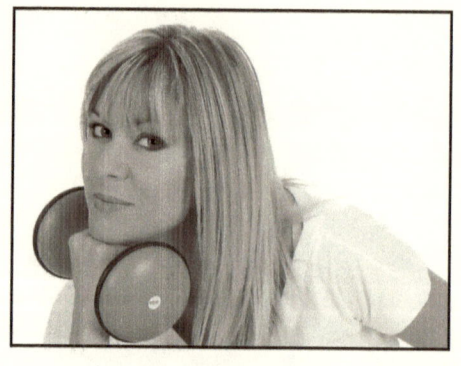

Try not to work out less than two hours prior to sleep because exercise at this time may prevent the body from receiving a good rest. Rest is important, and the body needs to rest thirty-six to forty-eight hours after each resistance training session. That is why I recommend twenty-one exercises that will target the whole body at one time, three days a week.

# The Benefits of Resistance Training

Resistance training decreases the risk for heart disease, hypertension, diabetes, cancers, osteopenea, osteoporosis, bone fractures, muscle tears, sprains, strains, arthritic conditions, such as osteoarthritis, rheumatoid arthritis, or the gout, gastrointestinal problems, fatty livers, dysfunctional gallbladders, stress, fatigue, insomnia, and IBS.

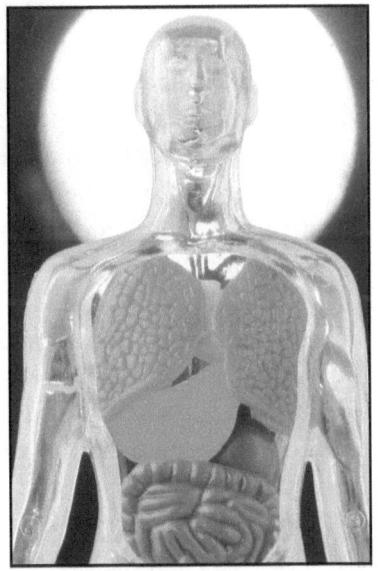

Everyday tasks will become easier to achieve. The brain will be sharper, and productivity will increase. Resistance training accelerates protein synthesis, which is the use of amino acids and proteins to repair and reinforce muscle fibers and increase the strength in the bones and muscles due to the calcium that is produced.

Most of this workout can be performed sitting or standing, and it also incorporates a floor routine (lying down).

The hardest part about working out is going to the gym.

# Gym Phobia

My fear of the gym began in my teens. I have always had a muscular build, and I carry extra fat in my chest and abdominal areas. Eventually I became fat all over my body. I liked being strong, but not fat, so at an early age I joined a gym. I walked in and noticed all of the mirrors; I didn't like the fact that I was out of shape, and I now had mirrors everywhere to remind me of that fact. The personal trainer was not very personal and set goals that were unattainable; I couldn't even finish the first workout. Someone who is out of shape and does not work out should not remain sore for a week or be expected to complete a workout for someone more advanced.

Each time before I headed to the gym, I would procrastinate about what I was going to wear. The girls that were already fit looked cute in their outfits, and I felt frumpy in my oversize shirt. I sweat a lot, and I was embarrassed because I become a hot, sweaty mess quickly.

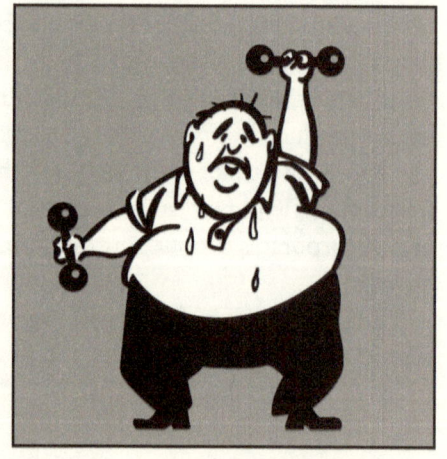

The classes I attempted left me discouraged because I was either not coordinated enough or couldn't keep up with the group because I had to rest or take frequent water breaks. The best parts of the gym for me became the whirlpool and Jacuzzi—and the eucalyptus room was totally cool. I spent hundreds of dollars on gym packages and personal trainers, and each time I had the same result. I noticed that each of us have a different level of endurance, and this is something that will increase gradually with proper training.

The advice that I received would work for someone who was already in shape and had a low body fat percentage, but not for someone that needed to burn fat, not calories. I eventually purchased a multi station gym, but I still wasn't sure what I needed to do to lose the fat. I tried to incorporate healthy nourishment choices at times, but I wasn't consistent. I lived in pain most of the time and suffered with problems like headaches, PMS, IBS, back pain, heel pain, acid reflux, anxiety, and depression. I was "tired of being tired," and I wanted to feel good.

The new lifestyle that I am committed to today includes "Black Jack" 21 three times a week and healthy nourishment choices daily. I feel great, and most of all, I am free from pain. I have made poor choices in my life in regards to diet and exercise, but it is never too late to reverse the curse and lower chances of further damage.

I hope to educate the public with this book because sometimes if a medical problem is explained in layman's terms, rather than medical jargon, a person may have a better understanding of the problem therefore be able to manage it better.

# Food Saboteurs

The items listed below can hinder fat loss or create fat if you are not careful with the amounts and frequencies.

Baked beans

Chips (potato)

Chocolate milk (premade)

Condiments

Energy drinks

Fat-free products like milk, salad dressing, peanut butter and mayonnaise

Fruit juices (eat fresh fruit and drink water)

Gravies

Hot dogs

Imitation crab

Instant flavored oatmeal

Omega 6; corn oil (increases inflammation)

Pretzels

Sodas

Sugar

Sweet tea

Yogurt with fruit added

Most fried foods

# Staples

The items listed below are convenient and can assist with fat loss and should be readily available to prevent hunger.

Apple butter

Blue corn tortilla chips

Brummel & Brown yogurt butter

Cheese

Clam sauce

Cookies

Crackers

Fish sauce

Grits

Lime tortilla chips

Marinades

Natural peanut butter/old fashioned peanut butter

Nutella (hazelnut chocolate spread), found in most grocery stores

Pompeii extra virgin olive oil

Regular salad dressings

Tortillas

Vinegars

Wheat germ

Worcestershire sauce

# Recipes and "Black Jack" Tips

### *Smoothies and Milk Shakes*

Ice (unless the fruit is frozen)
Any type of milk or water
Greek yogurt (plain or vanilla)
Optional items include but aren't limited to: natural
peanut butter/old fashioned peanut butter
cinnamon, vanilla, dark chocolate syrup, coffee, cayenne pepper
Fruit (any kind): blueberries, bananas, strawberries,
peaches, mangos, mixed fruit, etc.
*cayenne pepper speeds up the metabolism*
"Black Jack" tip: Most fruits can be frozen. For example,
peel bananas and place in Ziploc freezer bag.
Most fruits can also be found already frozen. Use within
six months for optimum nutrient benefits.
(A blender is required.)

### *Chicken Curry*

Cooked, deboned chicken, cut in chunks.
Place chicken in saucepan and one can of coconut
milk; add curry to taste, and stir.
Optional items: frozen spinach or broccoli
Serve over Basmati rice.
*Use more chicken than rice.*
"Black Jack" tip: If trying to lose fat, always eat
more protein than carbohydrates.

### Peel and Eat Shrimp

Shrimp with shell on
Marinate in Italian dressing add tumeric, paprika, salt
and pepper and garlic powder for fifteen minutes
Sauté in EVOO and butter (Brummel & Brown
yogurt butter) until pink or cooked thru
Peel Eat and Enjoy

### Shrimp and Spinach

Shelled and deveined shrimp
Sauté in EVOO and butter until tender and/or pink (depending
on type of shrimp), until the opaqueness is gone.
Add frozen spinach.
Serve over jasmine rice or your favorite pasta.
*Use more shrimp and spinach than rice or pasta
(try Seitenbacher all-natural pasta).*
*EVOO is extra virgin olive oil (try Pompeii Robust flavor).*
"Black Jack" tip: Marinate shrimp in Italian salad
dressing for ten minutes prior to cooking.

### Pasta Salad

Deveined, shelled, and cooked shrimp or cooked,
boneless, skinless chicken cubed
Cooked and chilled pasta
Vegetables
Italian salad dressing
Mix together; serve cold.
Any vegetables, such as cucumbers, broccoli, scallions,
tomatoes, peppers, carrots, celery, mushrooms, or onions
Optional items: cheese, olives
*Broccoli can be slightly cooked or blanched.*

### Quesadillas

Tortillas, any kind, any size
Deveined and peeled shrimp, lean chicken, beef, pork, or fish
Cook shrimp, fish, or meat in frying pan with EVOO and butter.
Add garlic, onions, or other vegetables and spices.
Optional items: cheese, rice, sour cream, guacamole, olives, beans
Place tortilla in frying pan, add preferred
fillings, and top with another tortilla.
Heat on low until warm; flip and warm other
side until cheese melts tortillas together.
Top with optional items

### *Experiment with Food and Spices*

I learned to cook with my Italian grandmother Yia-Yia and my
father who was Greek and Italian neither one of them ever measured
anything. This is how I know Cooking is not rocket science, and
it can be great fun and a master craft to improving your health.
Cooking at home allows you to know exactly what is in your food—if
you are trying to lose fat, then you don't need hidden fats and calories
that hide in food you do not prepare, and it saves a ton of money.
"Black Jack" tips: If you have prepared foods available all
the time and don't allow yourself to become hungry,
fast food can become part of the past.

### *Cinnamon Toast*

Bread
Butter
Cinnamon
Sugar
Butter bread, sprinkle with cinnamon sugar, and toast, broil,
or bake until butter melts and bread is a little crunchy.

### Cheese Toast
Bread
Cheese
Top bread with cheese or cheeses and toast, broil, or bake
until cheese is melted and bread is a little crunchy.
Optional items: basil and tomatoes

### Poached Eggs
Bread (toasted)
Poached eggs
Poach eggs and place over bread (toasted).
Optional: cheese on bread prior to toasting
*Eggs can be poached in boiling water, and
egg poacher trays are available.*
*Include fats, carbohydrates, and proteins with every meal or snack.*
"Black Jack" tip: It's great to hard-boil eggs ahead
of time and grab them as needed.

### Scrambled Eggs
Scramble eggs and cook in pan with butter
Optional items: cheese, frozen spinach thawed,
asparagus, onion, green yellow or red peppers
"Black Jack" tip: make a large amount and place in a crust or
pan and bake in oven 350 degrees until firm and fully cooked

### Egg Sandwich
Fry egg and place on bread or toast; add mayonnaise and/or cheese.

## *Too Awesome Soup*

In saucepan, simmer on low a few tablespoons
of EVOO, butter, and chopped garlic;
do not burn the garlic, or the soup will be bitter.
Add two to four quarts of tomato juice and stir.
Add fresh-squeezed lemon, optional pepper to taste,
cayenne pepper or hot sauce, and stir.
Add vegetables cut up in chunks, such as fresh eggplant,
zucchini, squash, peppers, onions, or mushrooms;
leave skin on the vegetables.
Bring to a boil, and then simmer until vegetables
are tender (usually about an hour).
*Cooking time will vary depending on the
size of your vegetable chunks.*
"Black Jack" tip: Add mushrooms about thirty minutes before serving.
Add a tablespoon of sugar per two quarts.
"Black Jack" tip: Sugar cuts down the acidity of tomato products and
lowers the risk of indigestion and heartburn, especially in tomato sauces.

## *Pears or Apples and Cheese or Old-Fashioned Peanut Butter*

Pears
Apples
Cheeses or old-fashioned or natural peanut butter
*A balanced snack and an excellent pick-me-up to
fuel the body for the next half of the day.*

## *Unsweetened Applesauce and Cottage Cheese*

One part unsweetened applesauce
One part cottage cheese
Mix together.
*It's an awesome snack.*

### Spicy Nuts

Any kind of shelled nuts; separate or mix them together.
*Try Seitenbacher nuts (all natural).*
Heat olive oil and butter in a pan over low heat; add nuts and stir.
Spread nuts on baking sheet and sprinkle with spices.
Optional spices:
Five spice
Garlic powder
Curry
Cinnamon
Sugar
Wasabi
Mrs. Dash products
Turmeric
Paprika
"Black Jack" tip: You control the amount of spices.
*These are a great snack, appetizer, and gift (include the recipe).*


### Avocado

Peel and slice or slice and eat right out of the
skin, topped with salt and pepper.
"Black Jack" tip: An avocado is best when still
a little firm but tender to the touch.
If shaken, you can hear and feel the seed moving


### Avocado Milkshake (contains coffee)

Ice
Avocado
Espresso or coffee
Sweetened condensed milk or any kind of milk
Vanilla
Blend together.
Optional: line cup with dark chocolate syrup
Top with whipped cream and dark chocolate syrup.

### Tomato and Cheese

Bread, slightly buttered (on the outside of the bread)
Sliced tomato
Cheese
Grill each side of this sandwich in a frying pan over low heat.

### Tomato Sandwich

Bread
Tomato (sliced)
Mayonnaise (regular)
Salt and pepper

### Wraps

Tortillas, any kind and size
Filling options:
Beans
Rice
Cooked fish, shrimp, lean meats, or poultry
Warm up the filling, place in wrap, and roll.
"Black Jack" tip: Mix together sour cream and
drained black beans and spread on tortillas.
Wrap, chill, and cut into slices.
Serve cold.
*A great appetizer or snack.*

### PB&J

Bread
Old-fashioned or natural peanut butter
Simply Fruit spread
Serve with a glass of milk.

## Hummus

one cup ground garbanzo beans or chickpeas
one tablespoon EVOO
Juice from one half of a lemon
Optional items: chopped, sundried tomatoes,
olives, crushed red pepper flakes
Serve with cracker or pita chips.

## Cream Cheese and Jelly or Salsa

Cream cheese and salsa or red pepper, jalapeno, peach, pear jelly, etc.
Serve with crackers.

# Examples of Foods to Eat

The items listed below can be better choices, not to mention convenient and should be readily available at all times to prevent hunger and cravings.

Beans

Bread

Cheeses

Crackers

Dark chocolate syrup

Eggs

Fig Newton cookies

Fresh and frozen fruits

Fresh and frozen vegetables

Greek yogurt, vanilla or plain

Lentils

Milk

Nuts (try Seitenbacher all-natural products; this company also carries gluten-free products available via their website Seitenbacher.com or in some grocery stores)

Nutter Butter cookies or your favorite cookie (remember, no deprivation and everything in moderation)

Old-fashioned peanut or natural butter (Smuckers is a great choice, with only one gram of sugar per serving)

Pastas (try Seitenbacher natural pasta)

Prunes

Simply Fruit spread

Tortilla chips (blue corn and lime)

Tortillas

Unsweetened applesauce

*Good daily nourishment choices* include fats, carbohydrates, and proteins with each meal or snack.

<u>Breakfast</u>

Fruit, veggies, cheese toast, eggs, cheesy eggs, tomato sandwich, egg sandwich w/cheese, smoothie or milkshake, BLT

*Eggs, apples, prunes, citrus fruits, and avocados keep you satisfied longer. Add cheese and fruit for a balanced breakfast that will fuel the body until the next snack or meal. See egg recipes

<u>Snack Choices</u>

Fruit and cheese, apples or celery, cucumbers and natural peanut butter/ old fashioned peanut butter or hummus, cucumbers with dressing, tomato, one half PBJ sandwich, one quarter avocado, vegetables with low GI values, milk and cookies, salsa and tortillas, smoothie or milkshake

<u>Meal Choices</u>

Shellfish, pasta salad, a wrap, one half PBJ or other sandwich, smoothie or milkshake, Greek salad with EVOO and vinegar dressing, rice, veggies meal, quesadilla, an appetizer, one half of any entrée, and all the recipes in this book

# How Much Should We Eat?

The nourishment choices that we make daily fuel our bodies differently. Healthy choices keep you feeling full longer and provide more energy to keep you awake and alert throughout the day. Eat frequent meals or snacks throughout the day that are balanced and include high quality or lean proteins, healthy fats, and carbohydrates like fruits and vegetables that have lower glycemic index values. The body requires a balance of nutrition to remain stable. The body, mind, and spirit all react to the nourishment choices we make. Portion control is something that has to be relearned. Once your stomach shrinks back to its original capacity, this will be easier to achieve, but it will take time, especially if it has been twenty years or more since you ate in a controlled manner. Remember that the stomach usually holds 1.75 liters, and it takes about twenty minutes after eating for the stomach to feel the state of fullness. The only thing a supersize meal is going to do for you is supersize your waistband!

# "Black Jack" 21 Resistance Training Program

These are full body resistance training exercises. Use dumbbells as needed.

### *"Black Jack" Program*

twenty-one exercises
two sets of each
fifteen repetitions per set

Start slow and gradual before using any weight for resistance. First, use your own body's resistance to become familiar with the exercise and the range of motion of each one, as well as your capabilities to achieve the full range of motion. Begin with one exercise at a time. "Black Jack" 21 can be performed using one side of the body at a time and alternating the extremities or using both sides at the same time. Try to aim for the twenty-one exercise circuit. A five-minute warm-up, such as marching in place and going through the motions of each exercise, will increase your oxygen levels. After the twenty-one exercises are completed, take five minutes to cool down by stretching the muscles, allowing the blood to settle back to the proper areas of the body. This decreases the risk of pooling of blood and prevents lactic acid from settling in the muscles, which causes swelling and pain due to the inability of the blood to circulate properly.

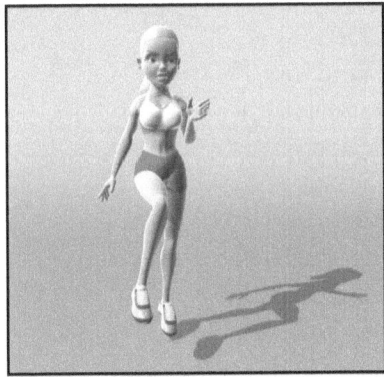 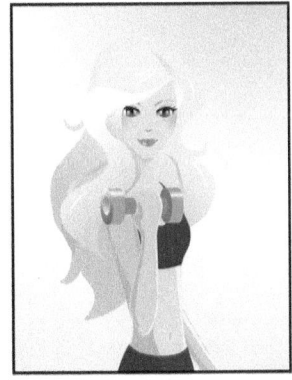

### *"Black Jack" 21*

fifteen bicep curls
fifteen shoulder presses
fifteen bicep curls
fifteen shoulder presses
fifteen hammer curls
fifteen upright rows

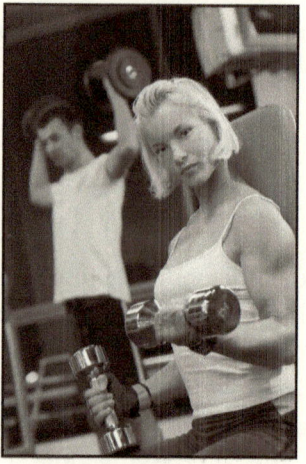

fifteen hammer curls
fifteen upright rows
fifteen front raises
fifteen shoulder shrugs
fifteen front raises
fifteen shoulder shrugs
fifteen lateral raises
fifteen dead lifts
fifteen lateral raises
fifteen dead lifts
fifteen squats
fifteen calf raises
fifteen squats
fifteen calf raises
fifteen tricep kickbacks
fifteen side bends
fifteen tricep kickbacks
fifteen side bends

(A side bend is a very small movement slightly bending
to one side at an approximate five-degree angle.)
*Incorporate dumbbells with the side bends for
optimal results and muscle tone/definition.*
fifteen tricep extensions
fifteen bent-over rows
fifteen tricep extensions
fifteen bent-over rows

*Floor Routine*

fifteen flyes
fifteen shoulder presses
fifteen flyes
fifteen shoulder presses
fifteen cycling
fifteen floor crunches
fifteen cycling
fifteen floor crunches
*Incorporate a dumbbell by placing it over the upper
abdominals for floor crunches for added definition.*
fifteen leg curls
fifteen leg raises
fifteen leg curls
fifteen leg raises
fifteen pelvic tilts
fifteen pelvic tilts
*Incorporate a dumbbell by placing it over the lower
abdominals for added muscle tone/definition.*

A push-up requires a person to lift ten times their own body weight and
is a good exercise for someone who has a strong core it is also true with
planks. This is not an exercise for a beginner; a person who is out of shape,
over fat, or overweight and cannot lift even their own body weight one
time. A sit-up may cause injury, especially for someone with back problems.
Trying to balance on a ball with a free weight is just dangerous! A better
alternative is an abdominal crunch for the upper abdominal muscles, a
pelvic tilt for lower abdominals, and side bends for the obliques. These
exercises will strengthen the abdominals, which will result in a strong and
stable core and improve posture.

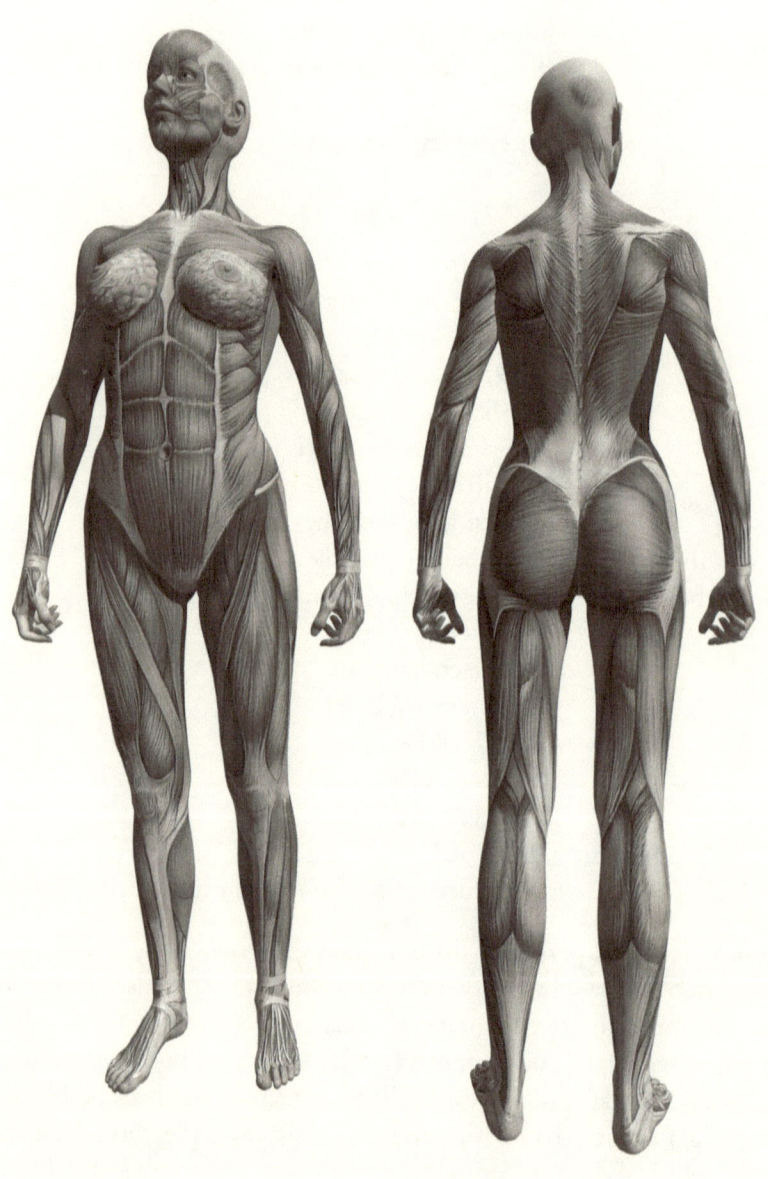

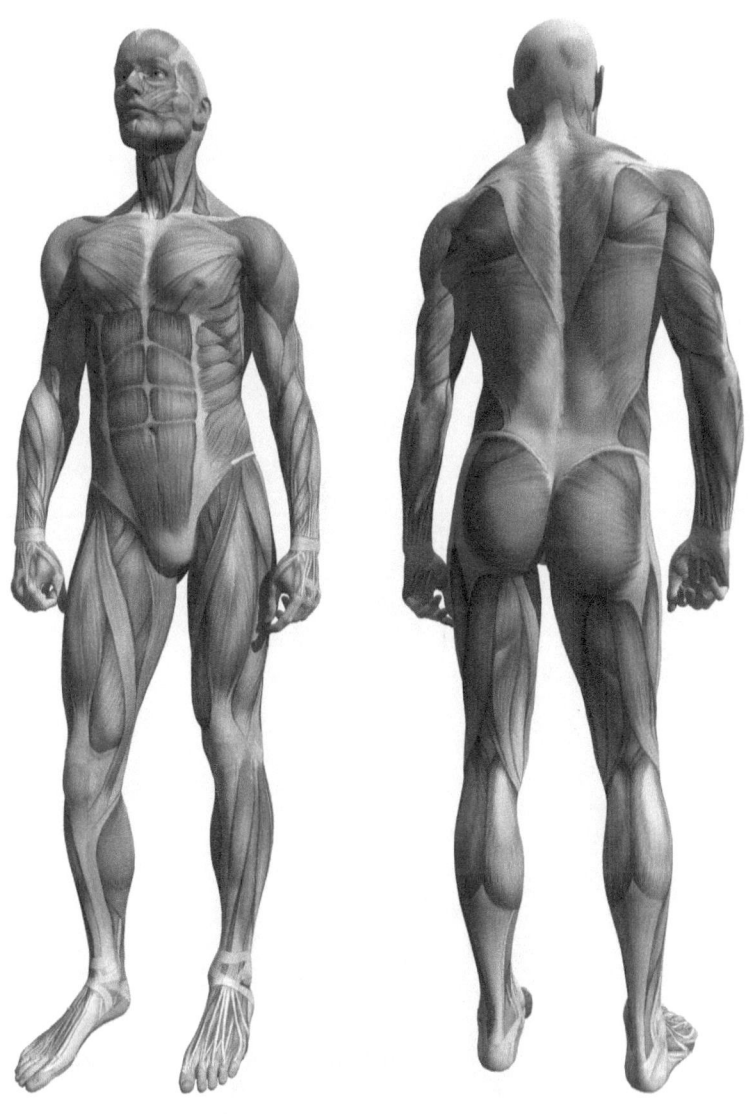

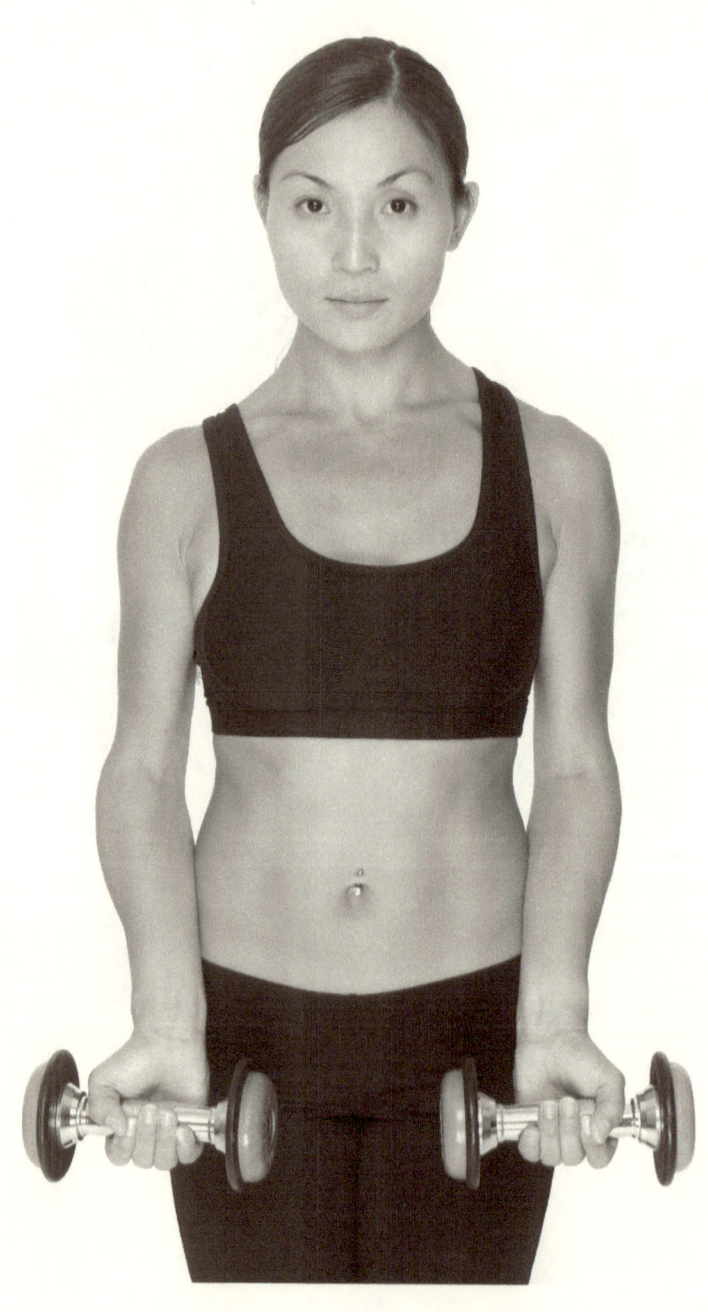

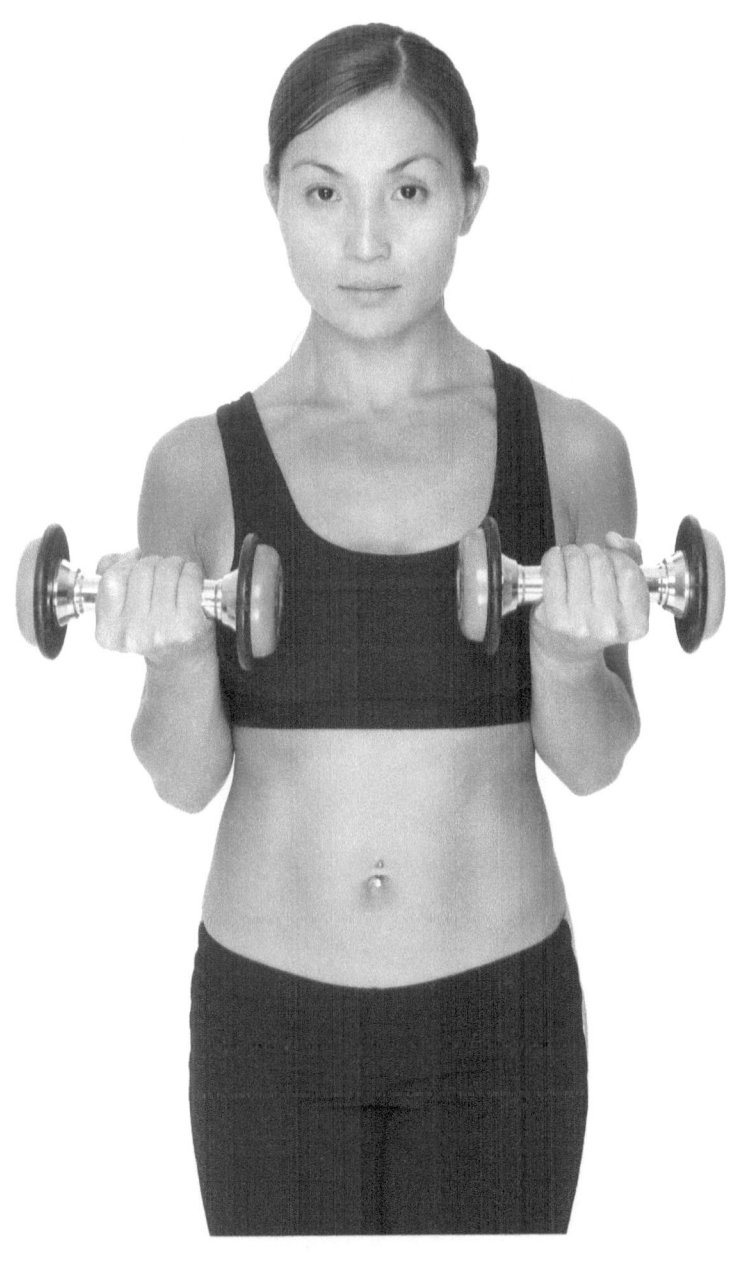

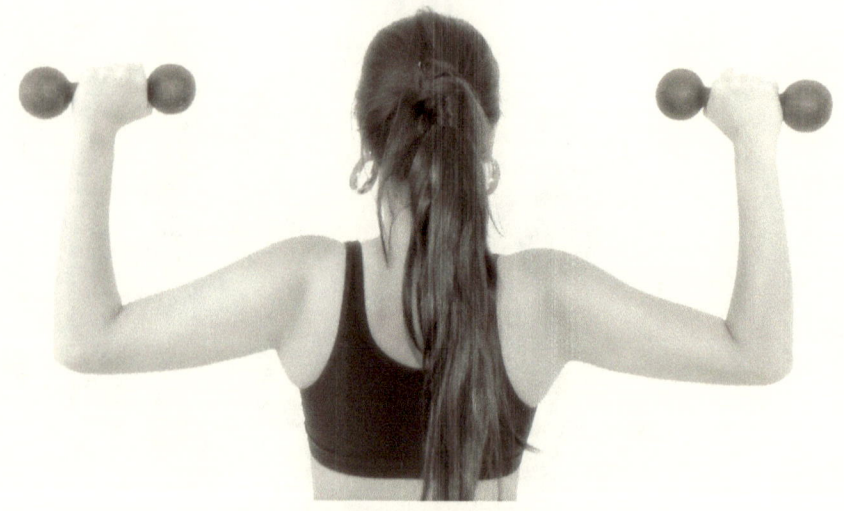

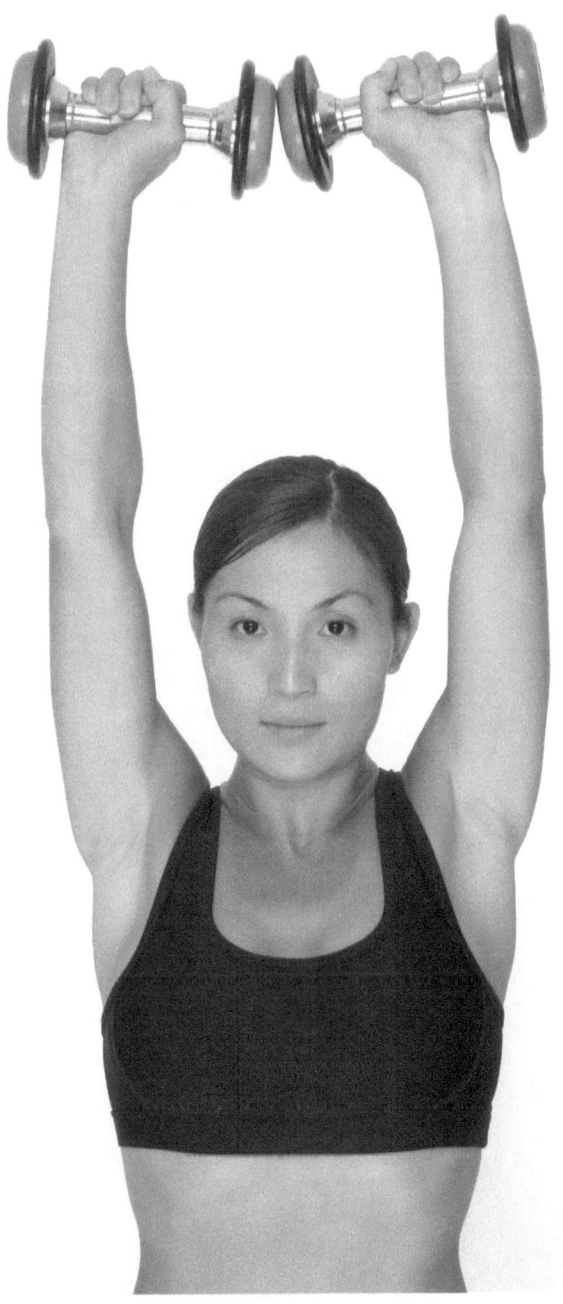

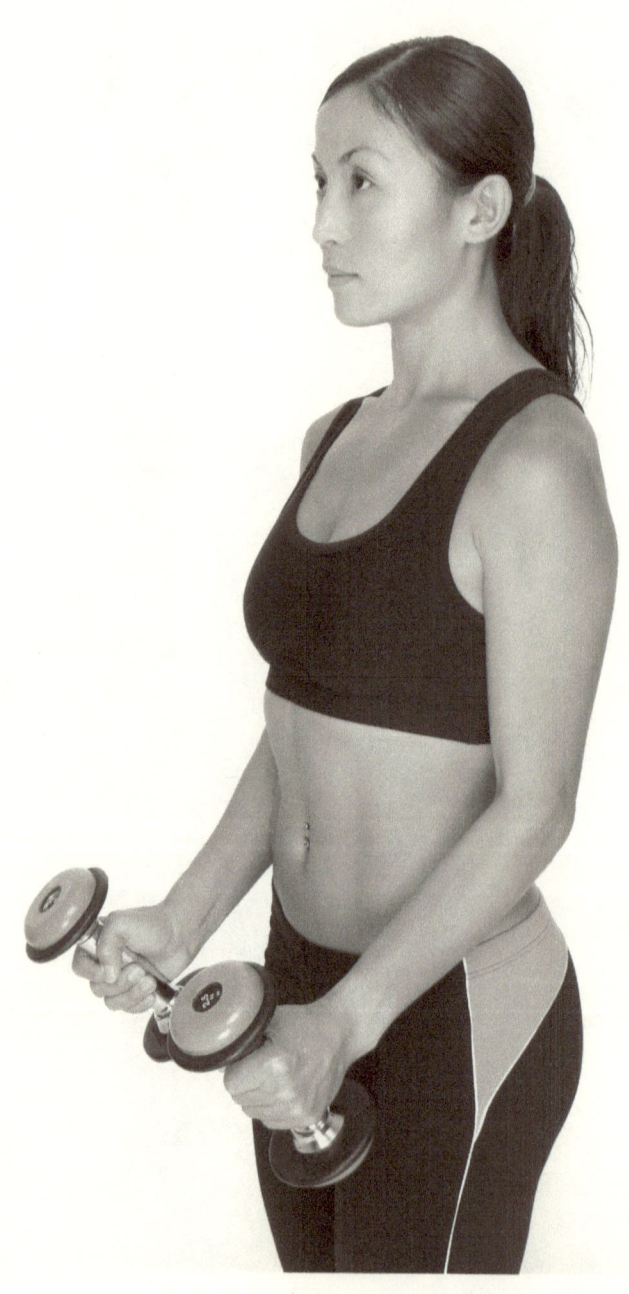

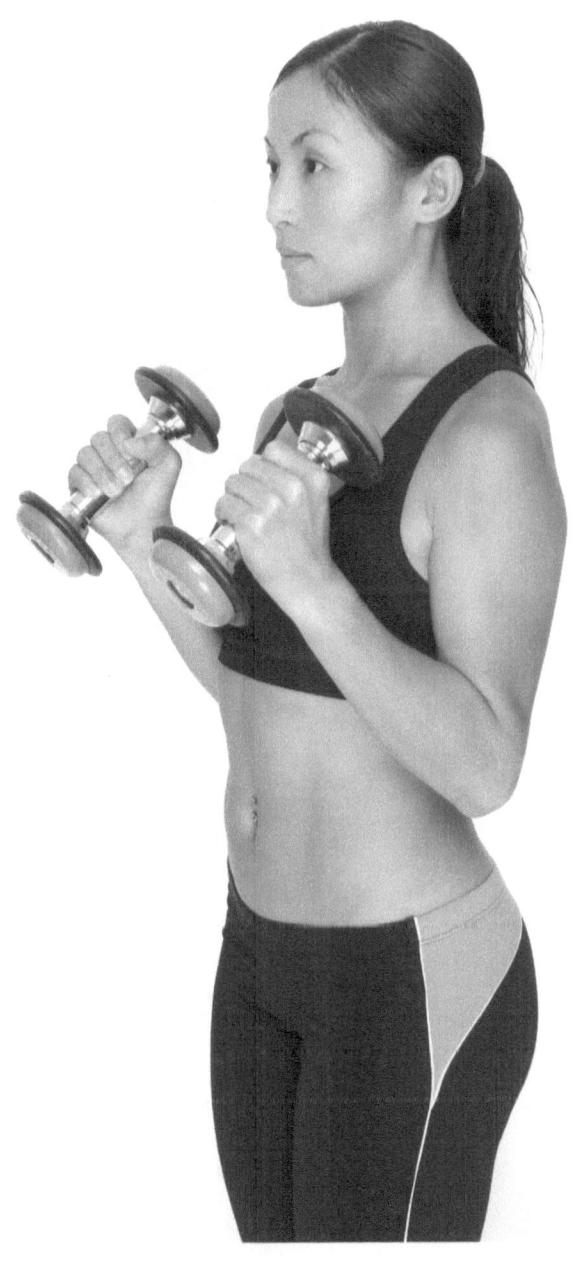

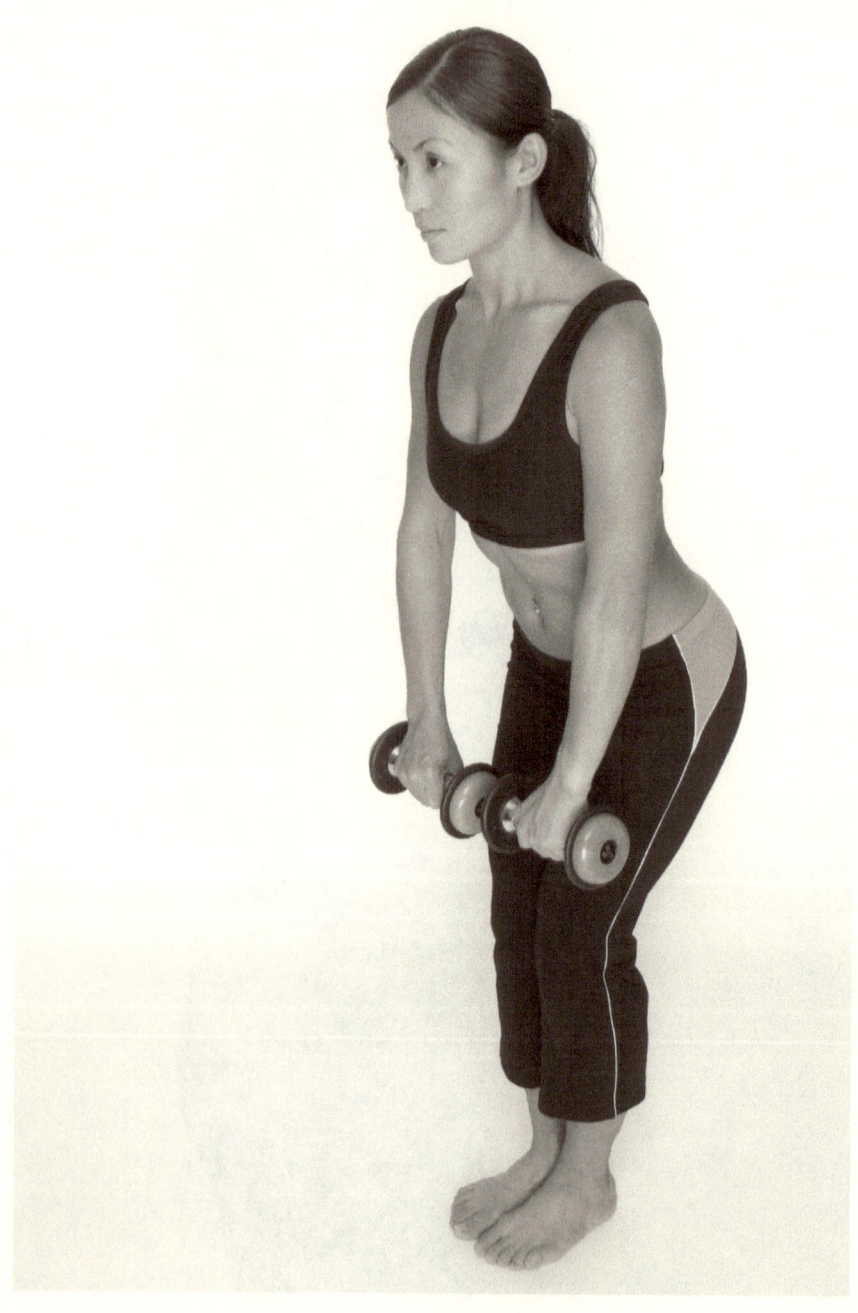

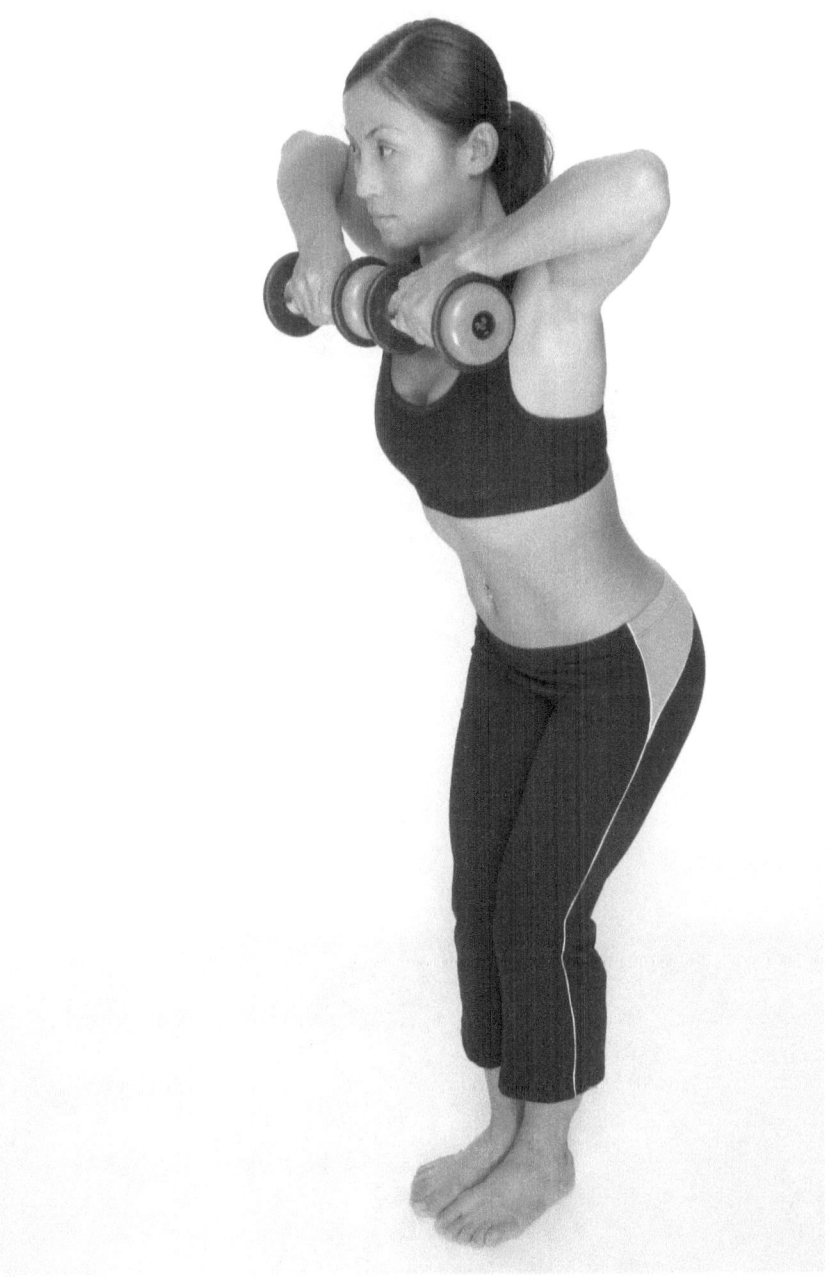

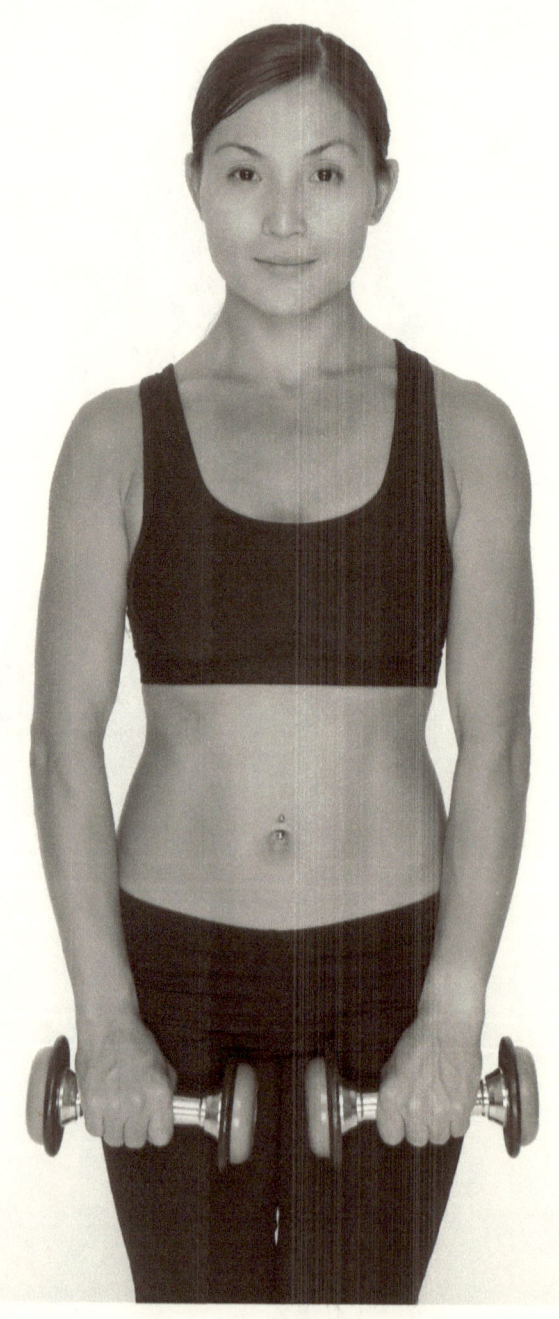

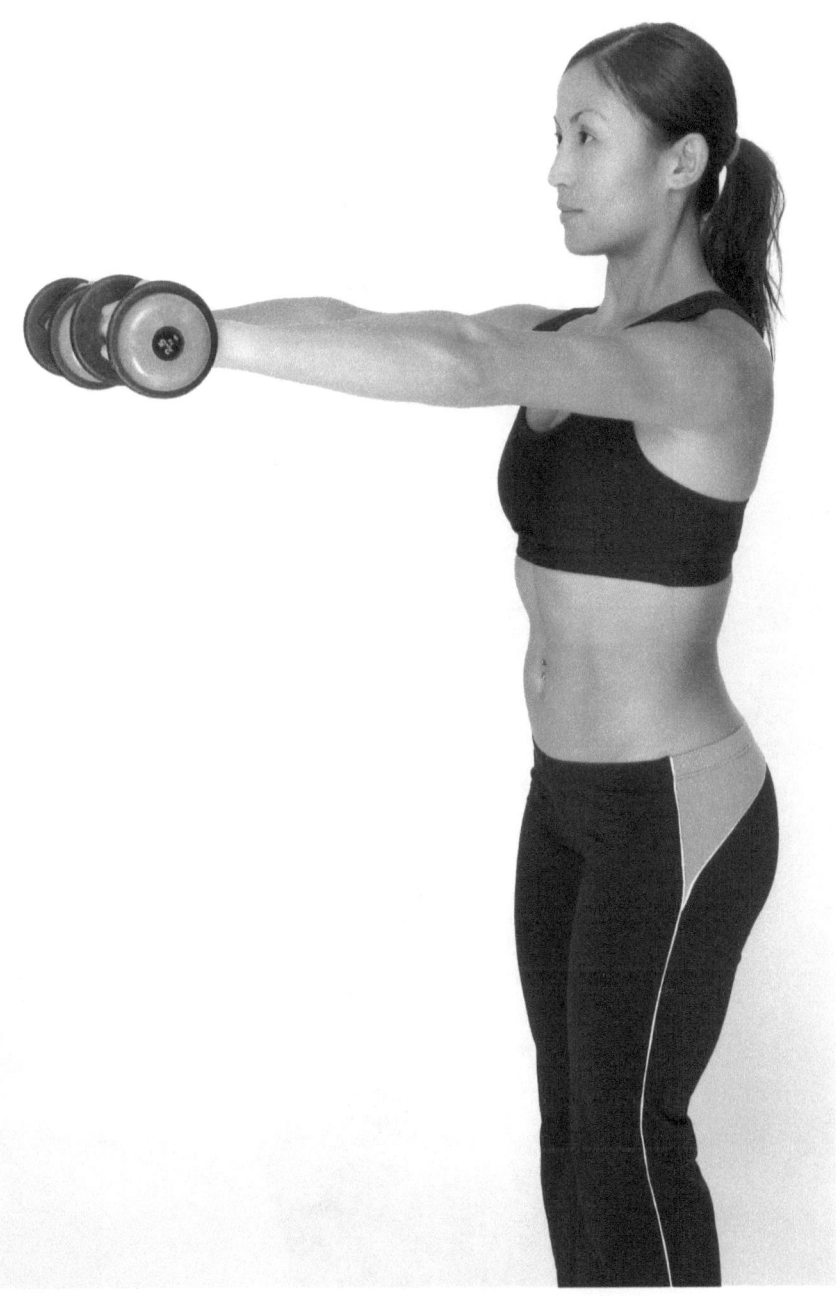

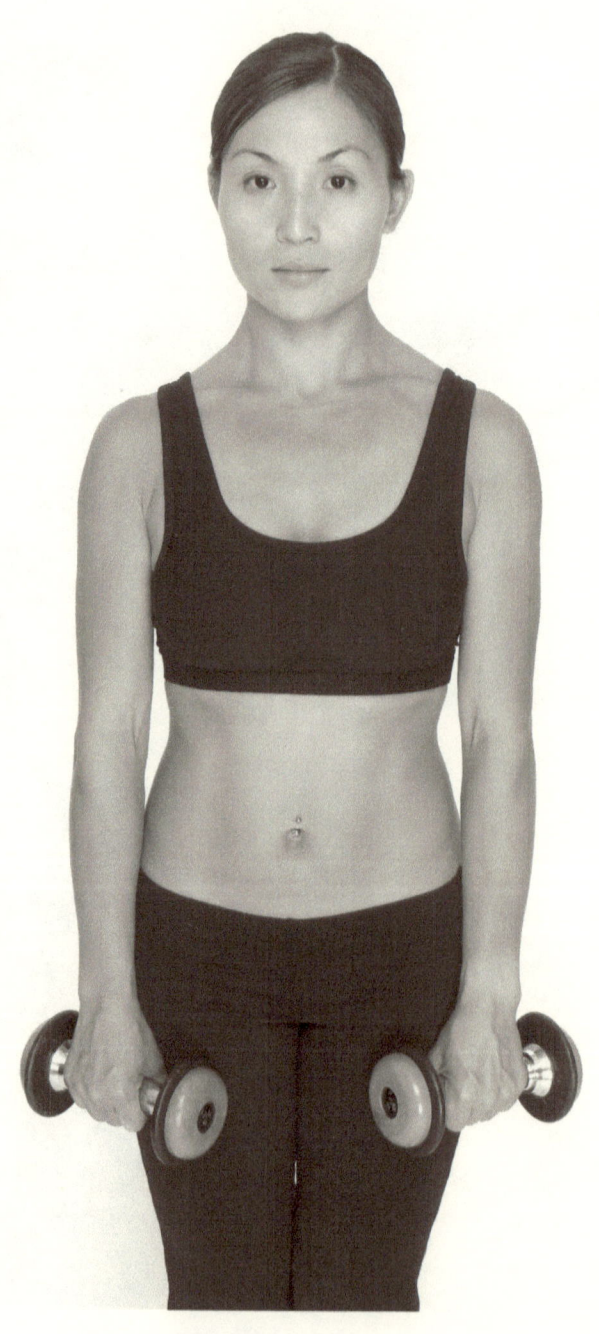

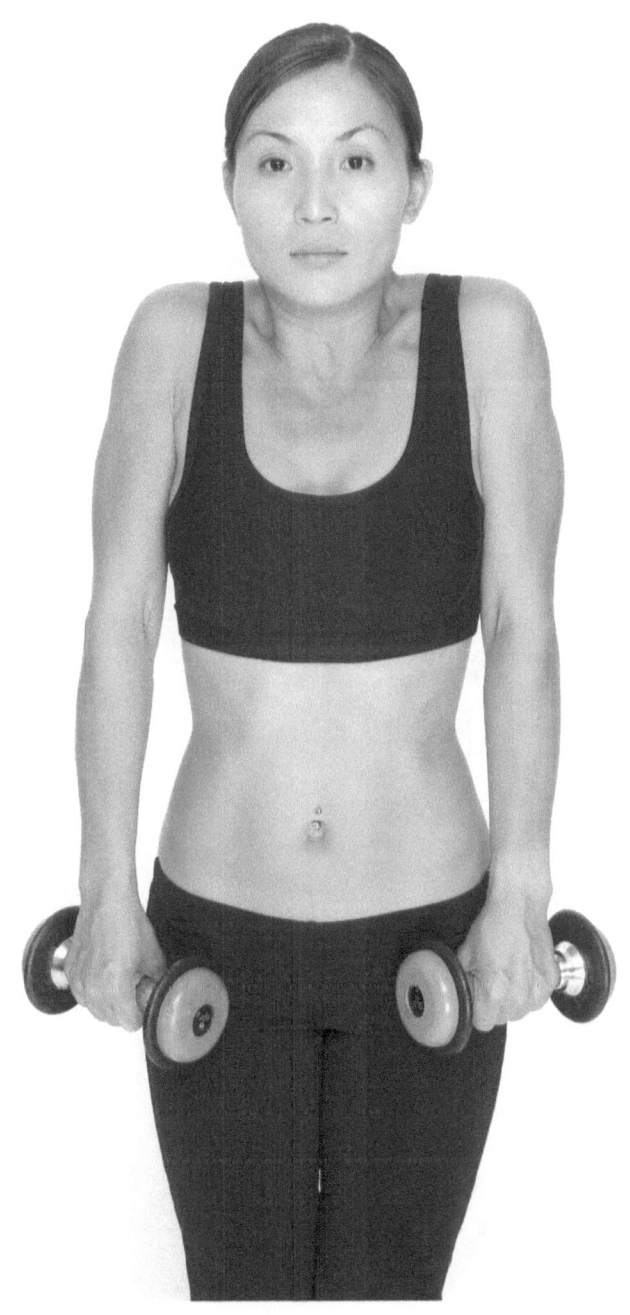

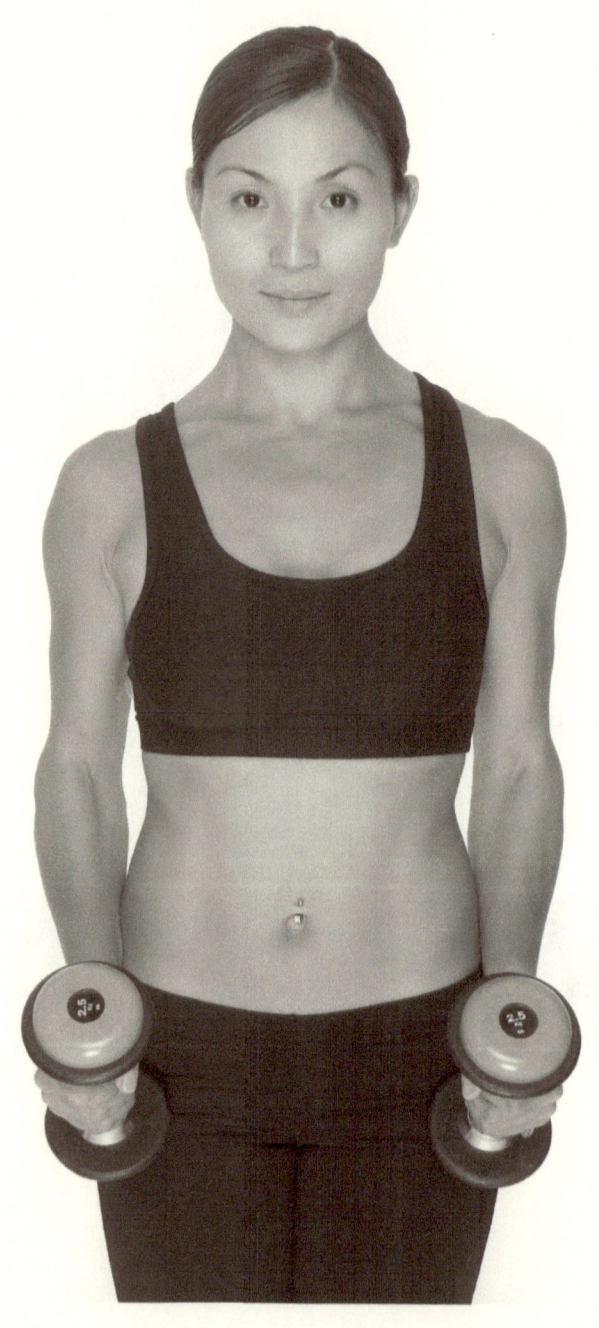

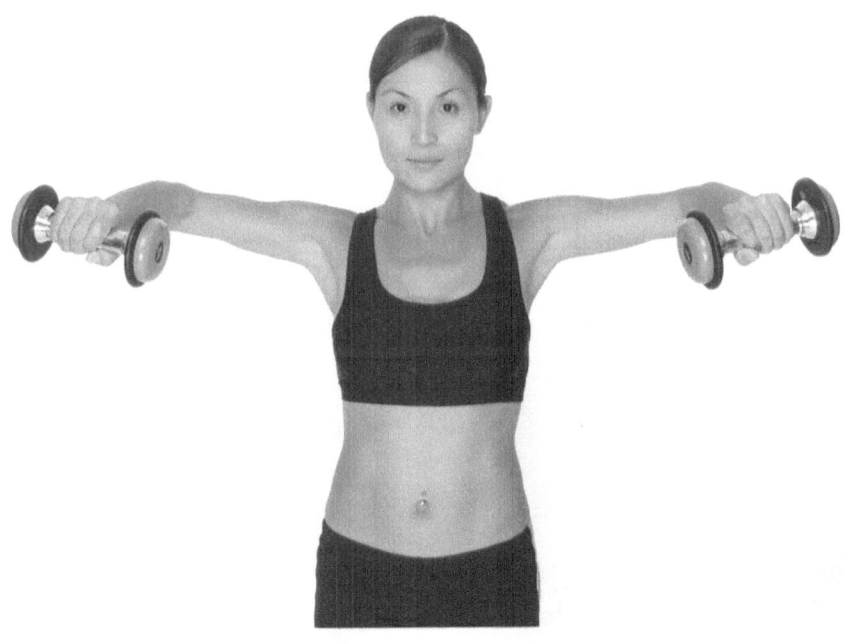

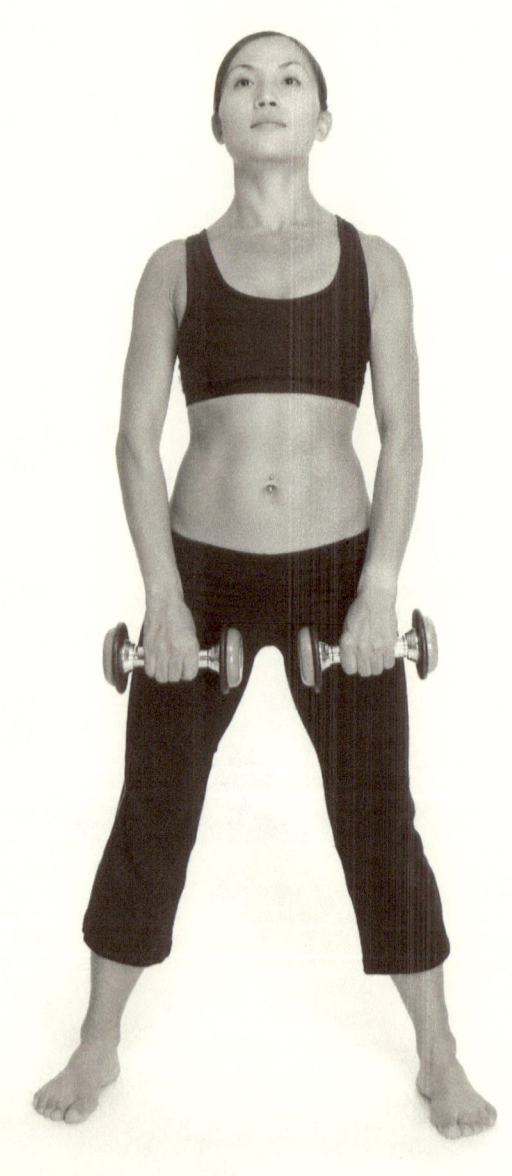

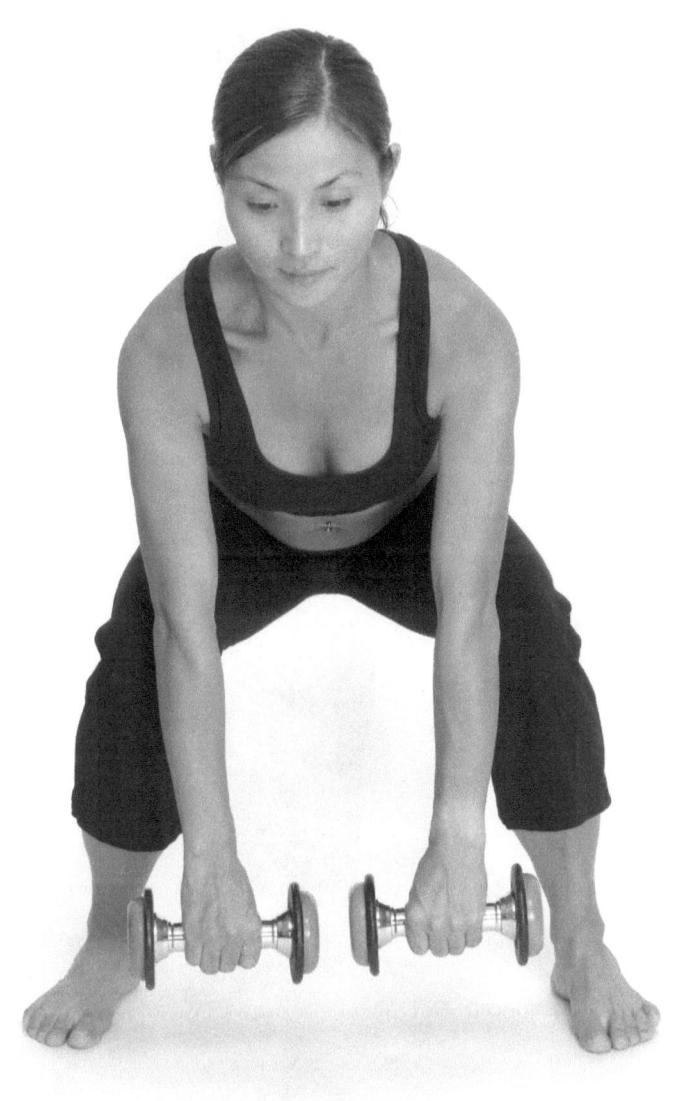

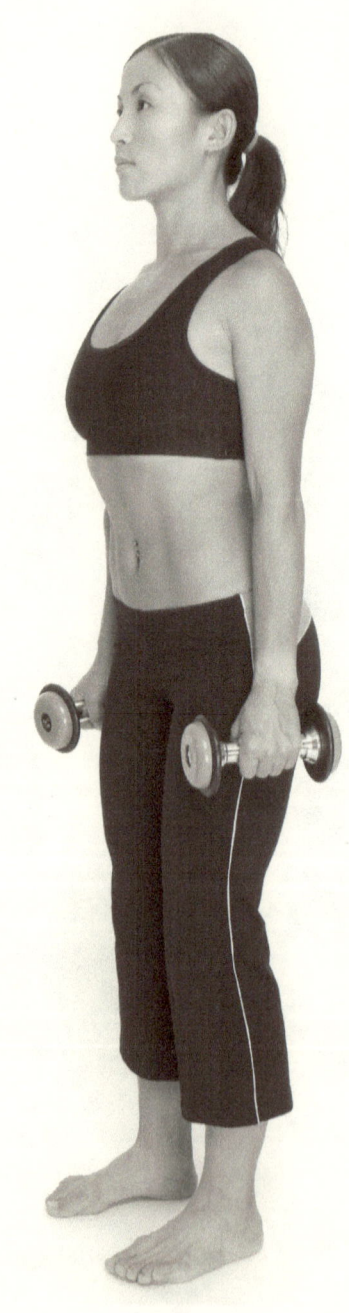

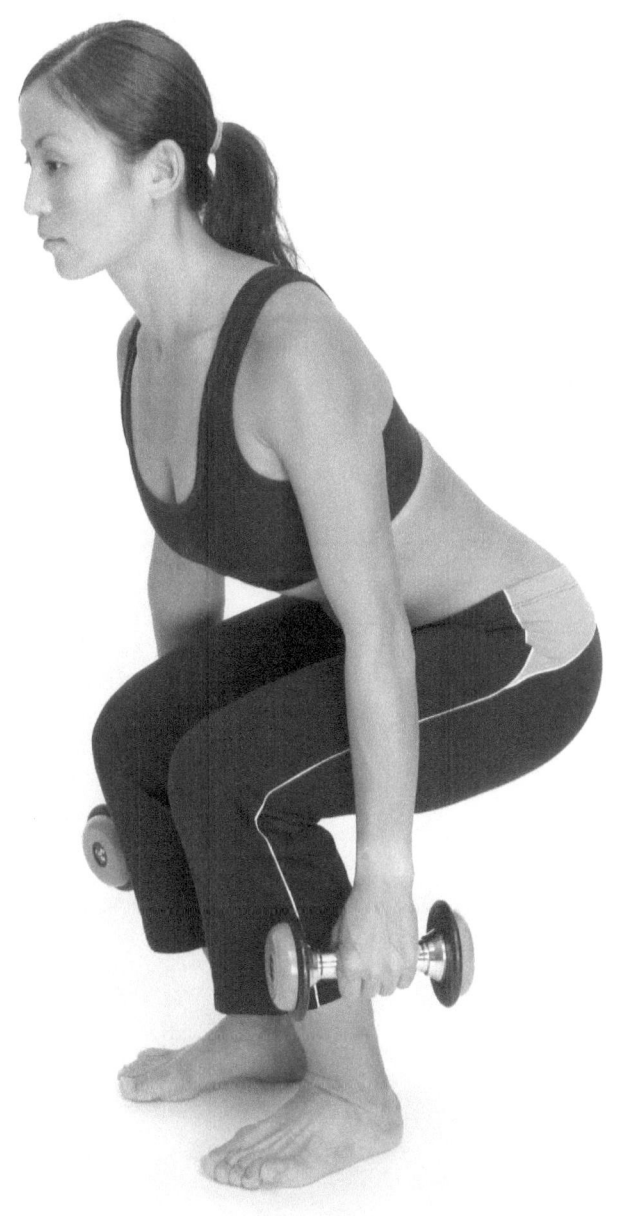

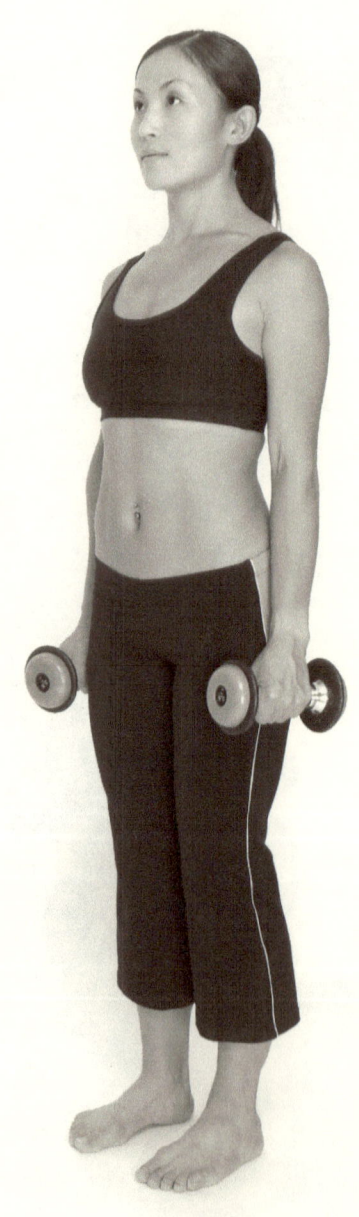

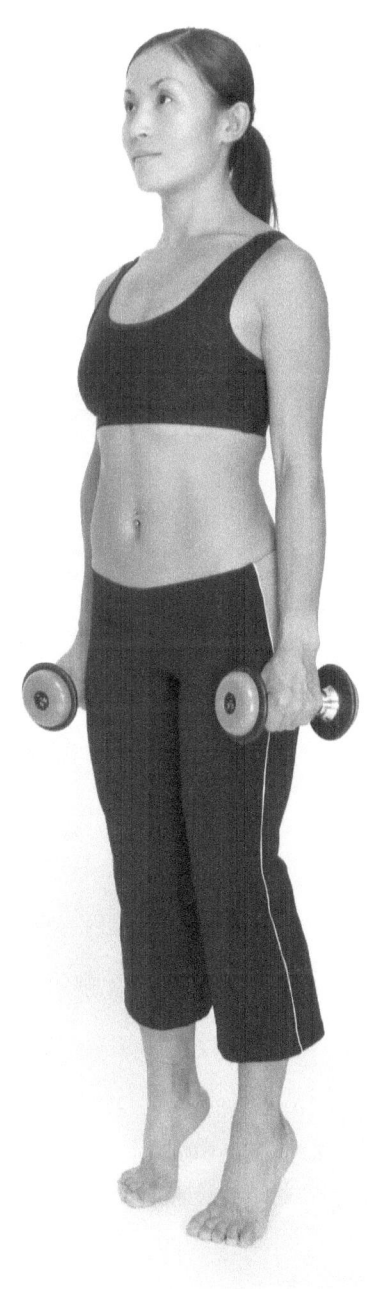

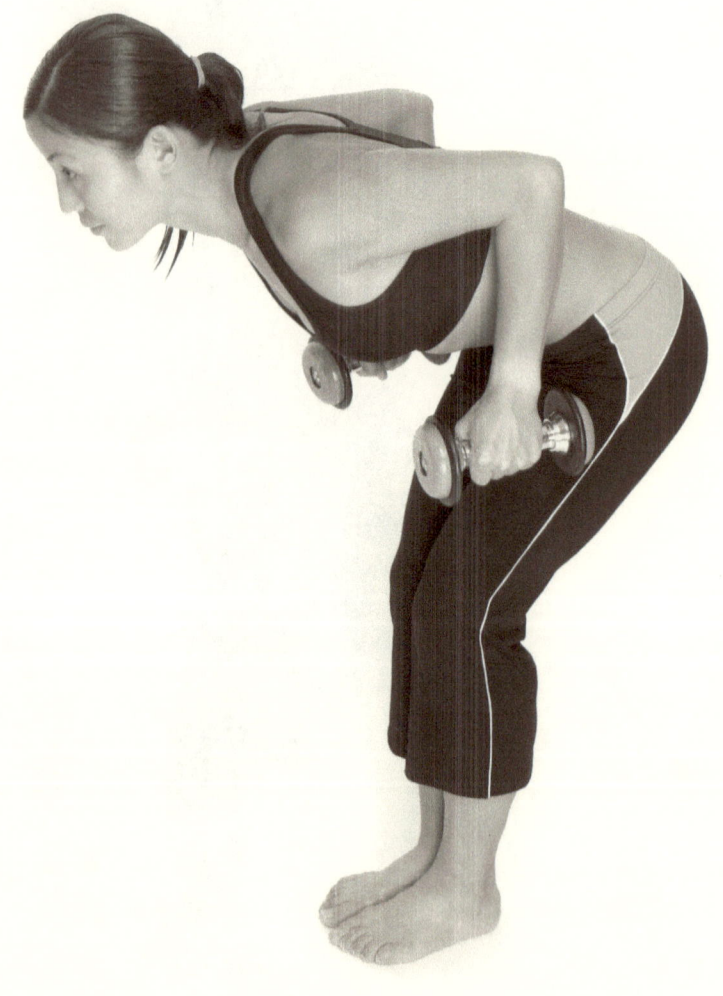

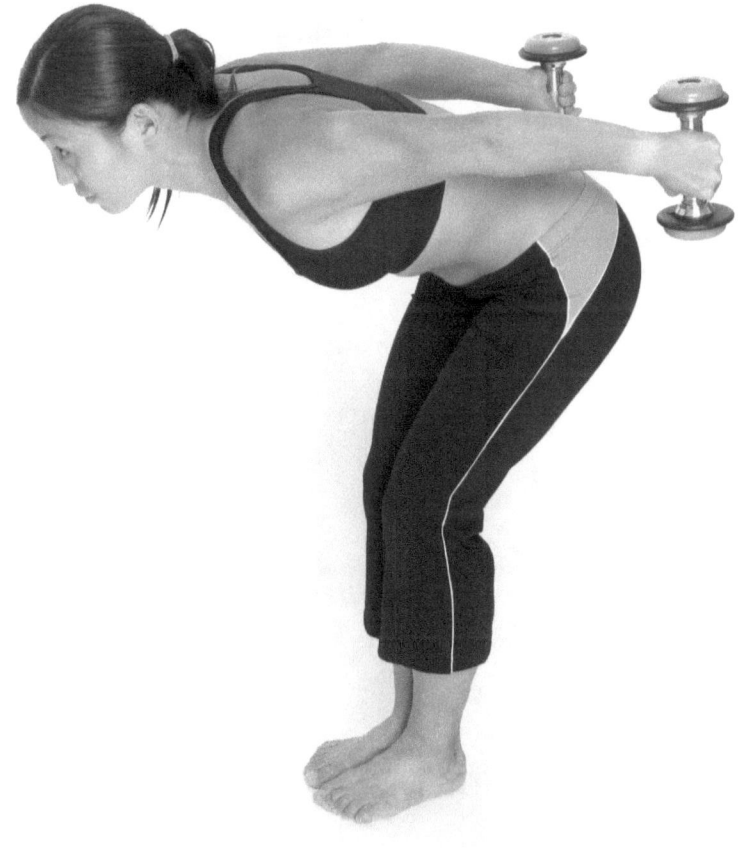

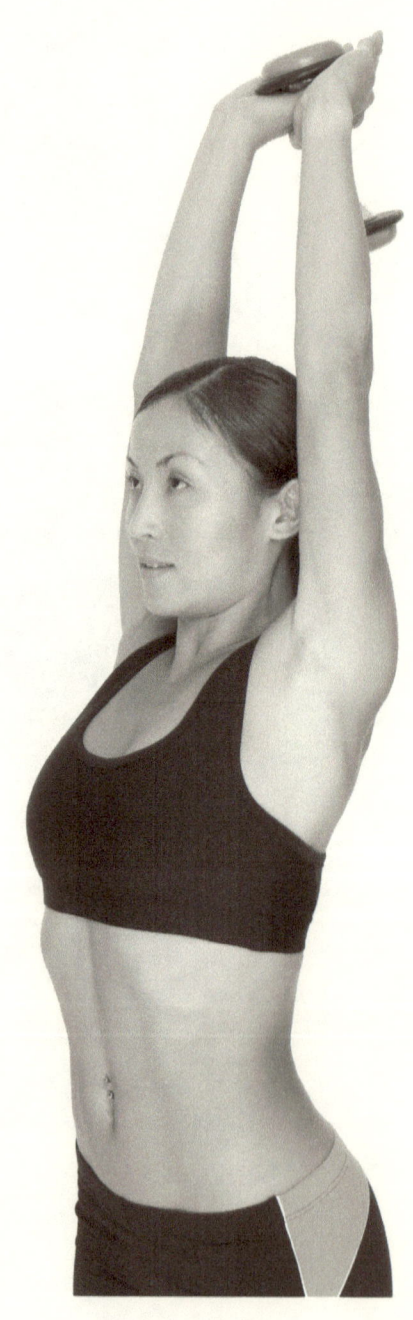

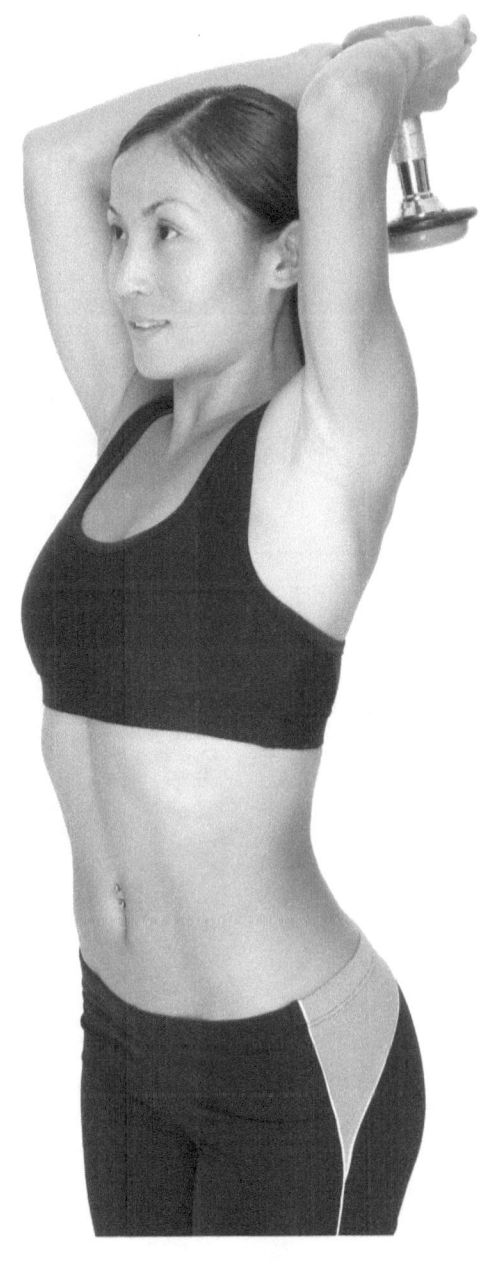

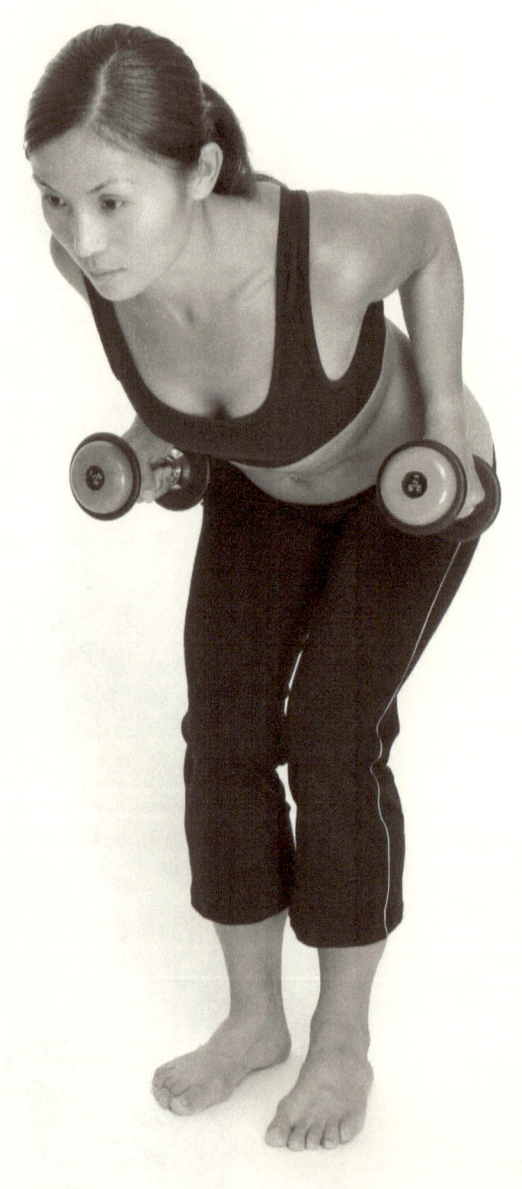

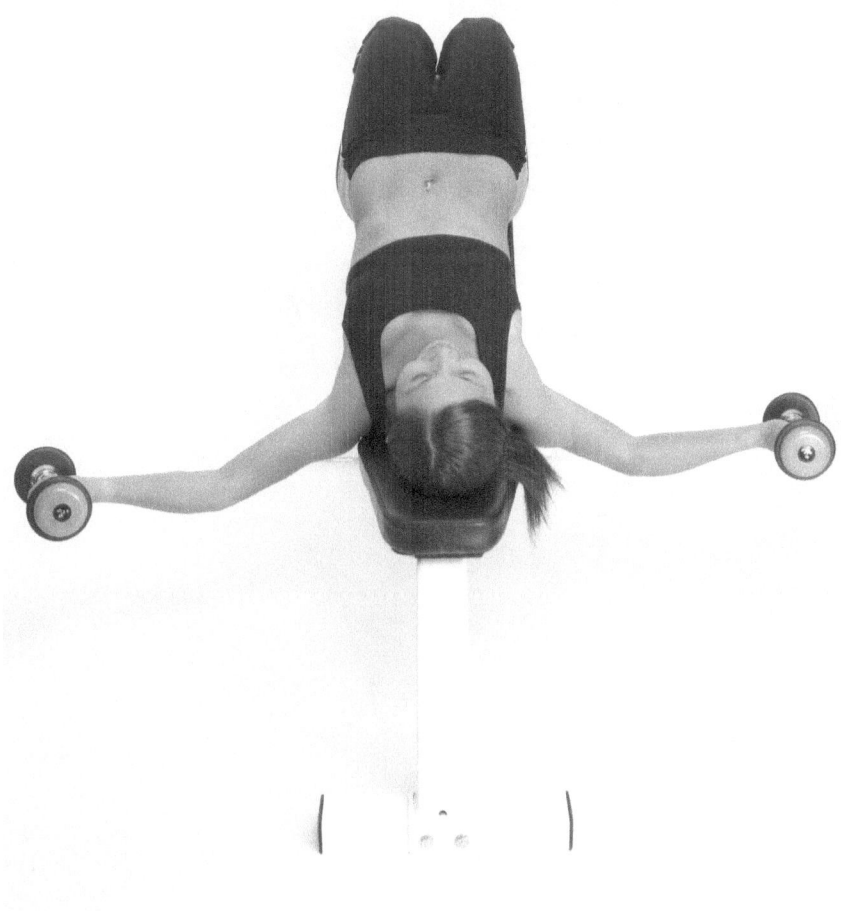

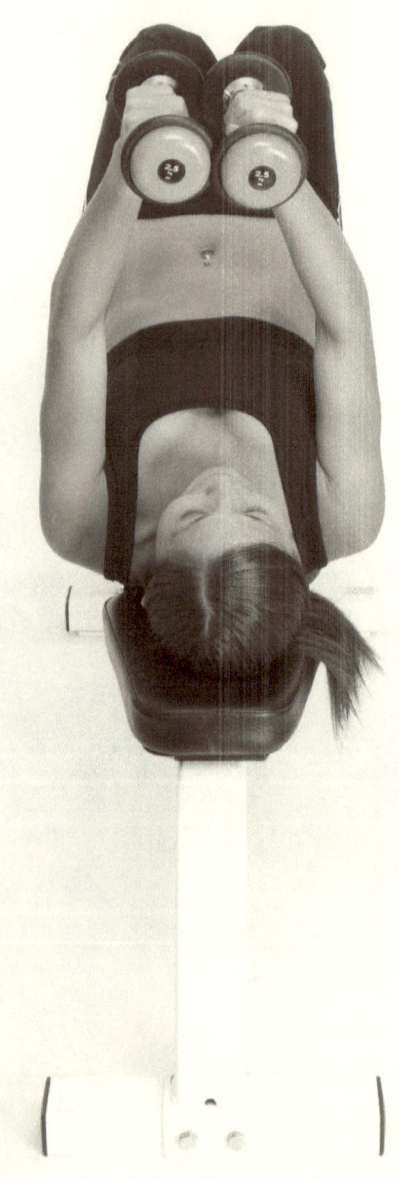

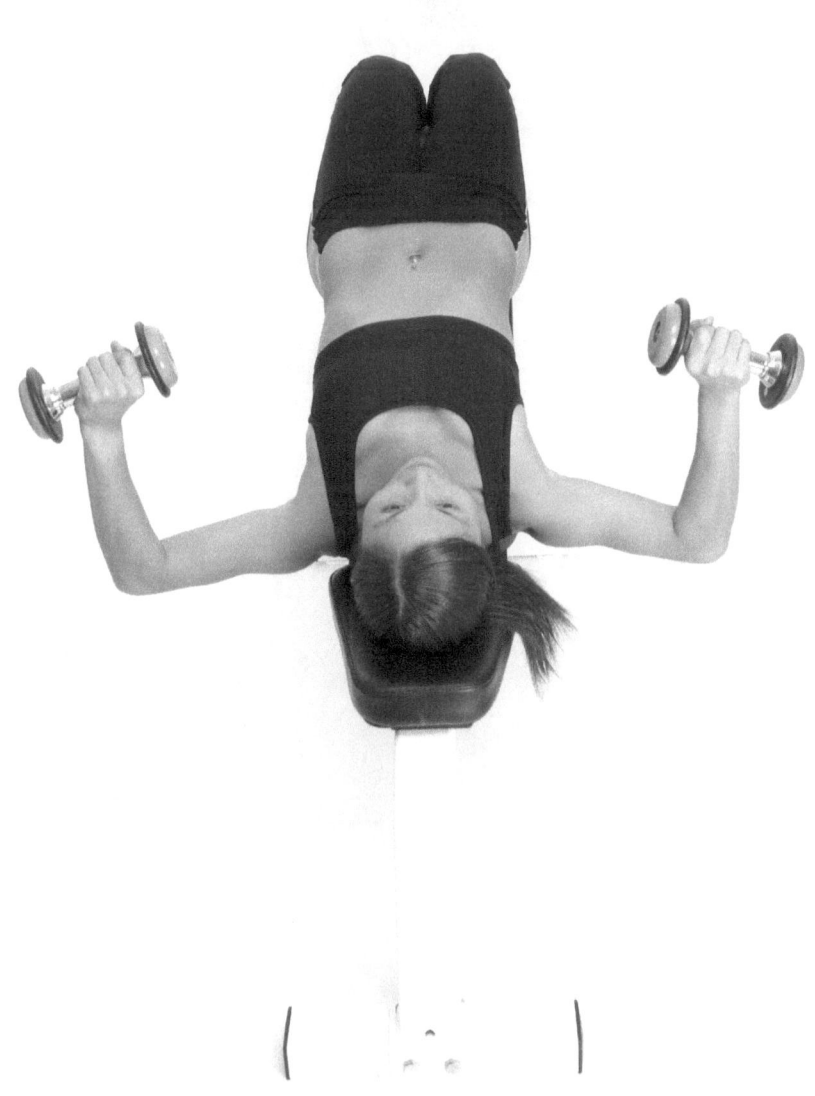

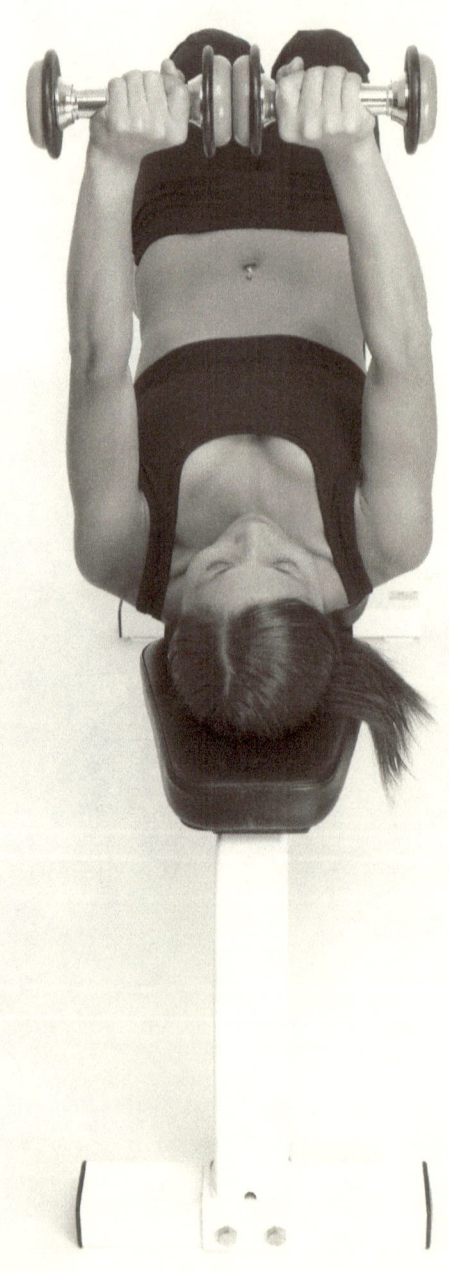

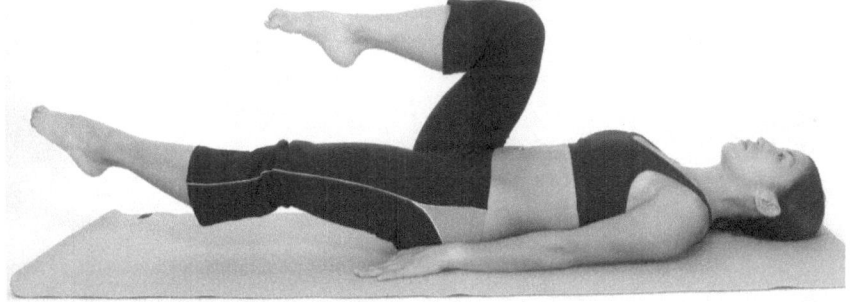

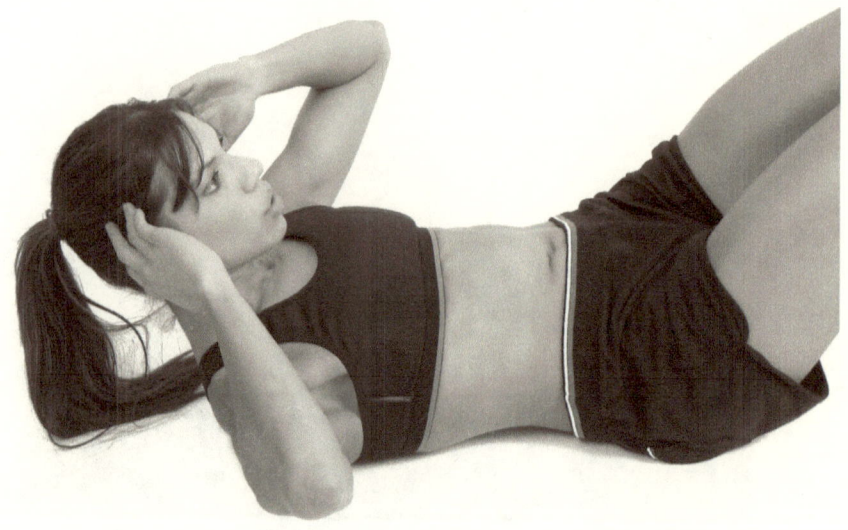

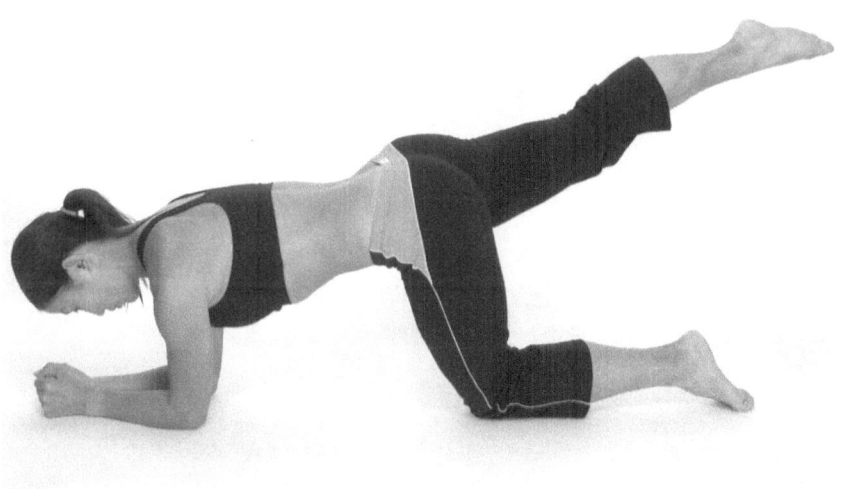

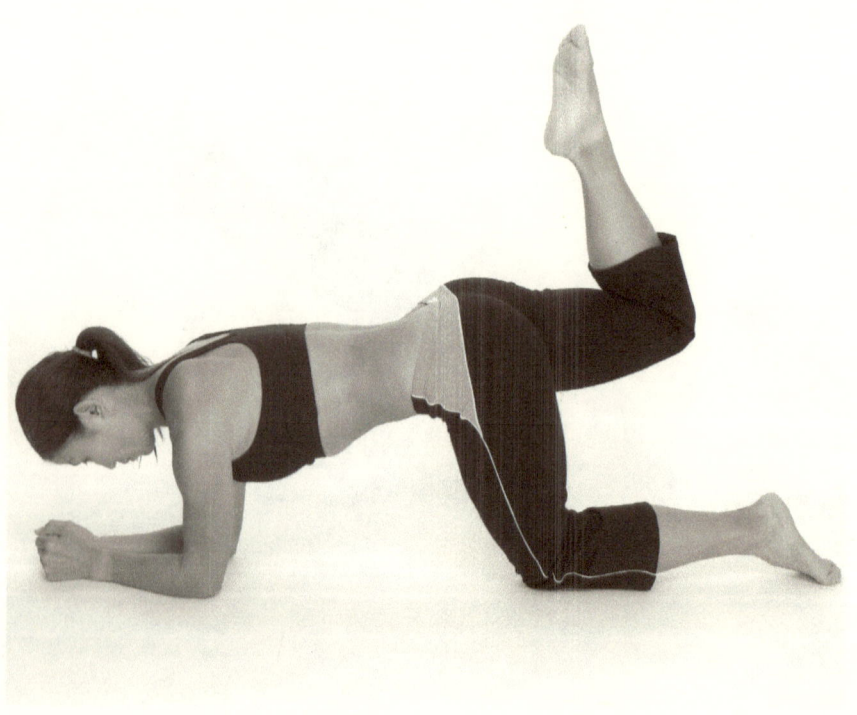

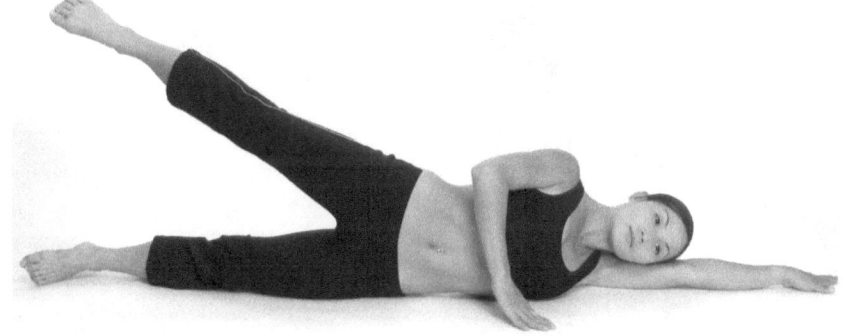

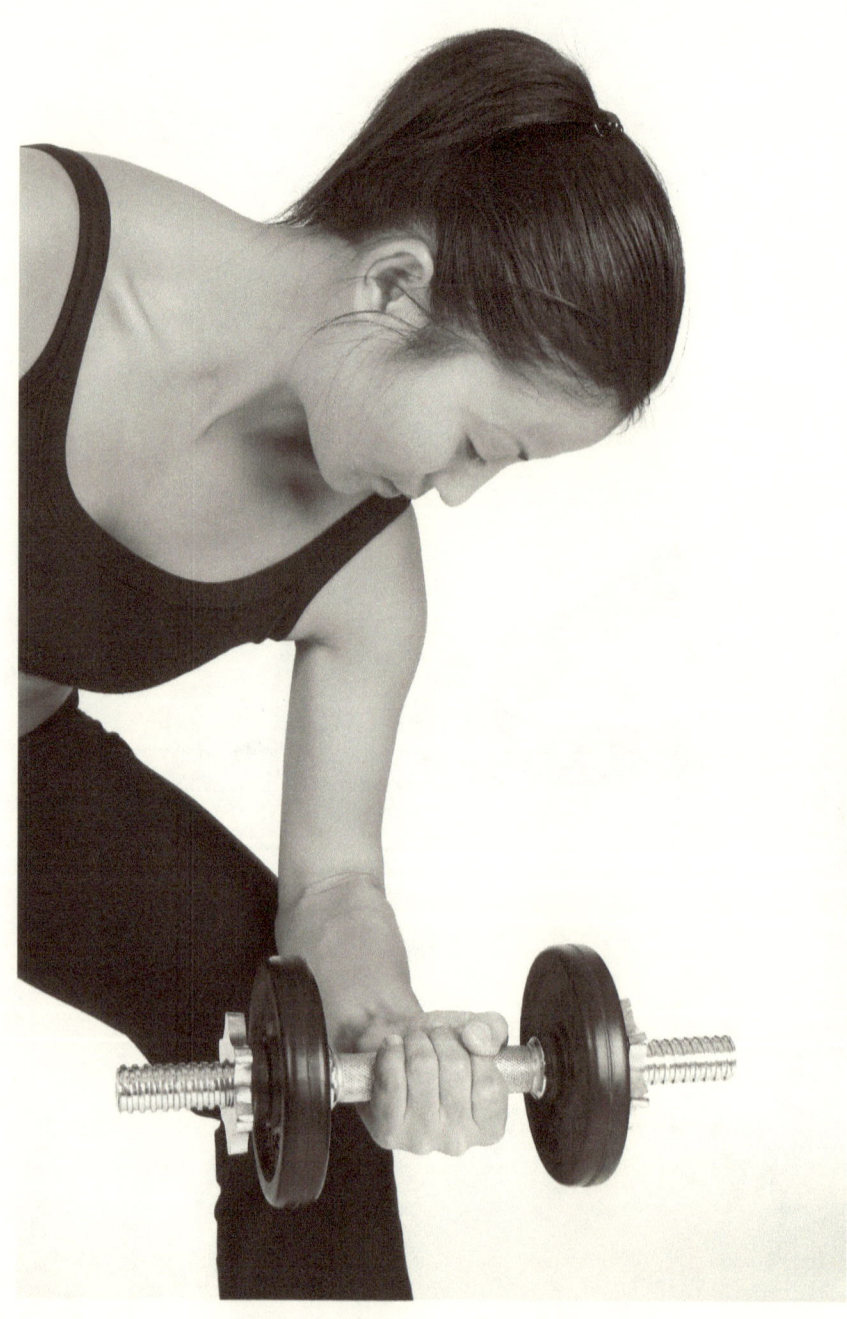

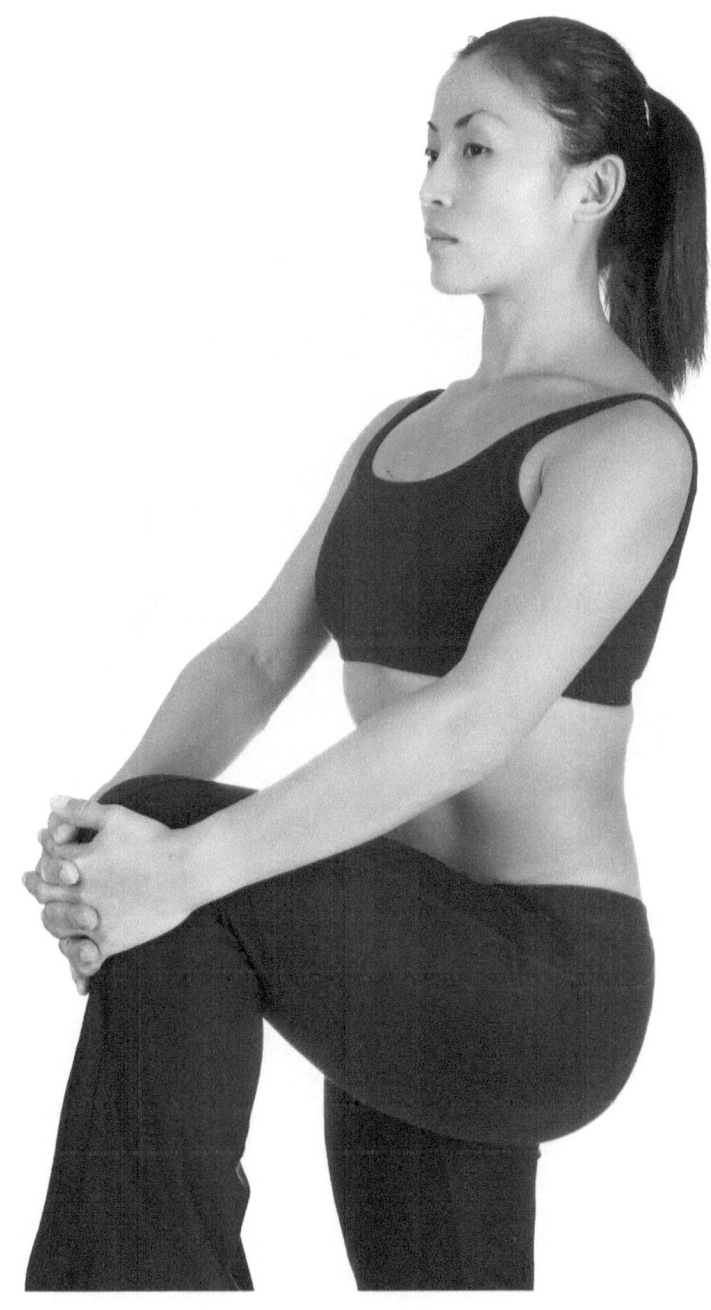

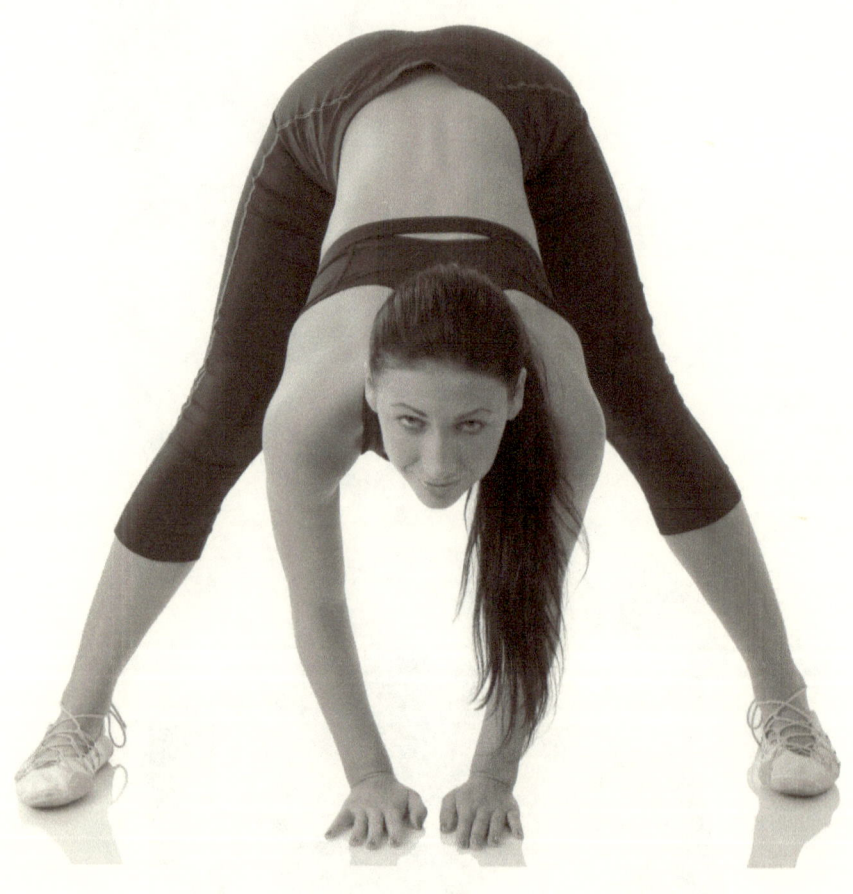

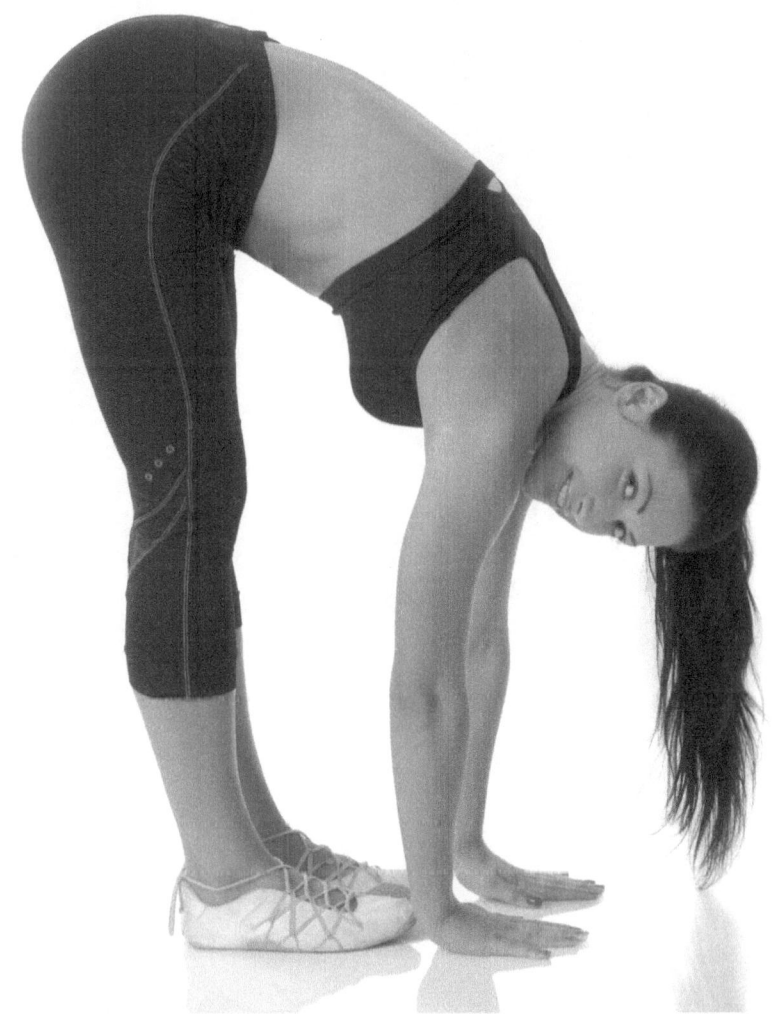

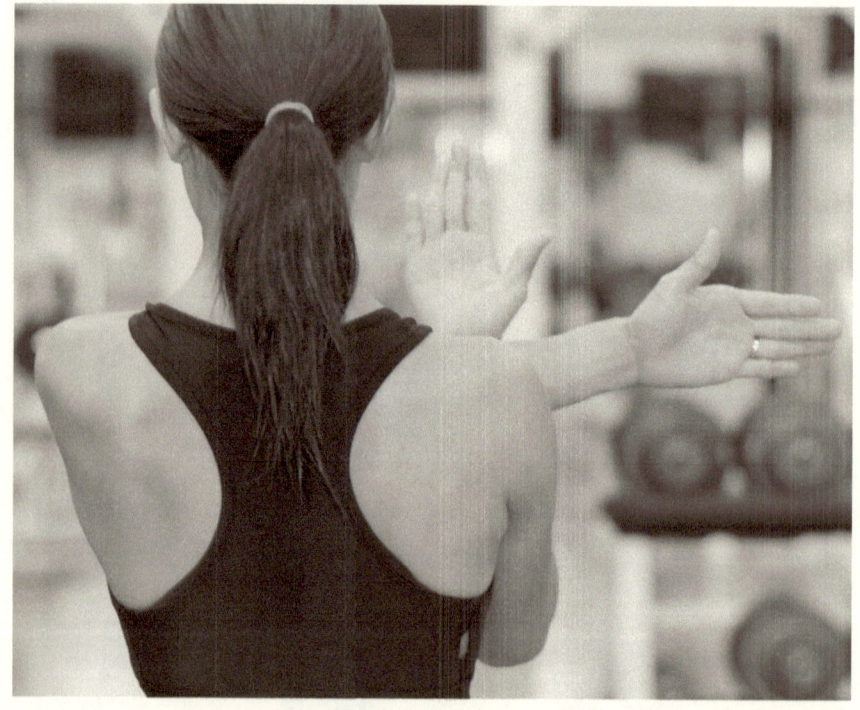

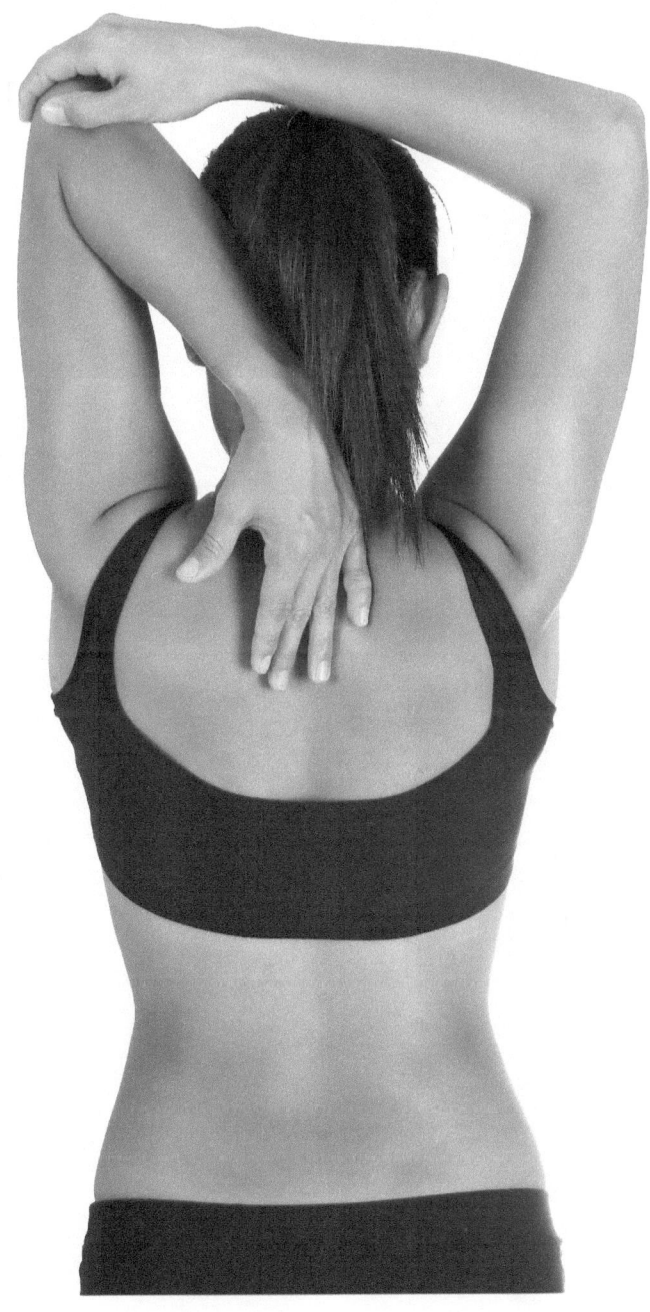

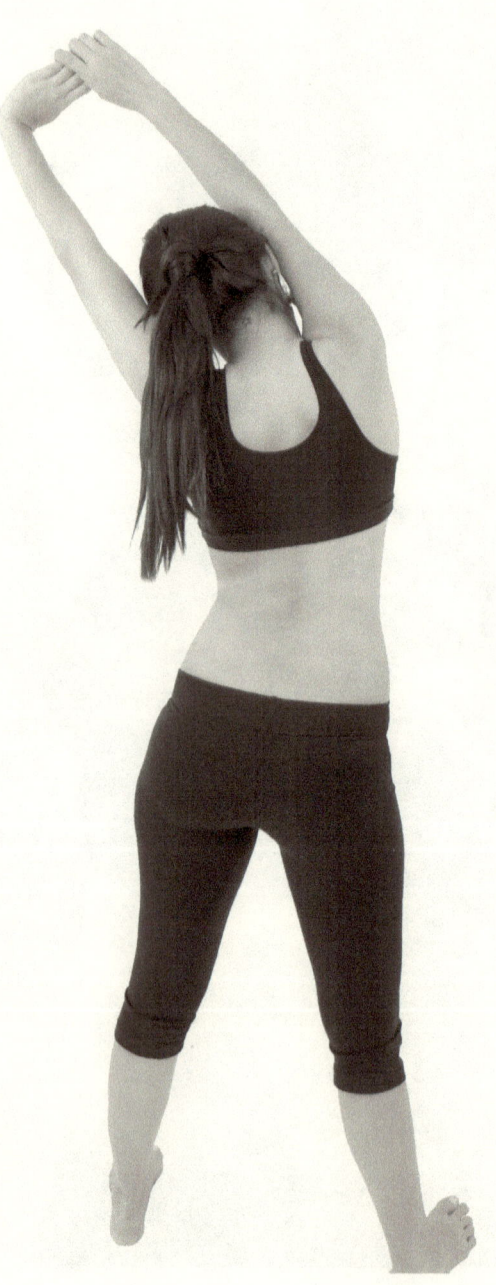

# Autobiography

Growing up, I was an active child. We lived in the country on a lake, I rode my bike all the time, and we always had a swimming pool. As soon as I reached puberty, I started to notice more fat appearing over my chest and stomach. Several years later, I noticed fat appearing on my upper arms. Over time, the fat increased all over my body, and I became less active. I was uncomfortable and lived with some kind of pain almost daily.

I worked in health care most of my life, and I observed firsthand the risks that being over fat can cause. I also watched my father suffer with heart disease due to unhealthy nourishment choices, lack of consistent exercise, and smoking.

After many failed attempts for a fast, easy way to lose fat, including fad diets and diet supplements, I contemplated weight augmentation surgery, but luckily I have a low pain tolerance and I chickened out every time because of the experiences I've had working in healthcare I've seen the single surgery that turns into multiple surgeries due to scar tissue, further injury or weight bearing on a particular muscle or joint, complications, infection etc...

I noticed that many health care employees are fat and unhealthy just like me, and we were increasing our own risks of becoming the patient instead of the caregiver.

For years, I tried to incorporated healthy nourishment choices daily prepare meals at home and decrease the number of times that I went out to eat or had fast-food items. I had a multi-gym for a long time, many years later I purchased a resort-size treadmill. For two years, I power walked three or more times a week and covered approximately five to ten miles a week. Because I was burning calories, I lost a couple inches and some weight, but I still had fatty deposits. The more I worked out, the easier it became to make these changes but I felt exhausted after this type of work out and not energized. I remember how I loved feeling strong when

I tried to resistance train and I had the multi-station gym at my disposal in addition to several free weight/ dumbbells.

I realized that some of the foods I thought were healthy are not, because what I needed was to lose fat! I finally learned about the glycemic index value and how it relates to the nourishment choices that we make every day.

After four years of conducting over fifteen thousand pre op interviews for anesthesia at an orthopaedic surgery center, I noticed that most of the patients were uneducated about their own health.

I incorporated a fitness and nutrition program that includes healthy nourishment choices daily that will fuel the body and provide energy. It also includes "Black Jack" 21, twenty-one resistance training exercises that will produce lean muscle mass and burn fat. This resistance will be different for each individual and it will depend on the strength of the muscle or joint that is used.

This combination has stabilized my hormones and my mood and blood sugar levels, which has decreased my cravings and desire to binge. It has also decreased my aches and pains and has allowed me to lose the fatty deposits, decreasing my risk for health problems and increasing my life span. In less than a year, I have transformed my physique; the fat literally melted off and still is gone, and I am four sizes smaller than when I began. I am strong! I feel great! My hair, skin, nails, and teeth are in better health than ever before, and others tell me that I look ten years younger than my real age!

I encourage anyone who has ever tried to lose fat to take the "Black Jack" to Lose Fat challenge and get *your* body and groove back! And I commend anyone who can shake a weight for one minute, not to mention six minutes!